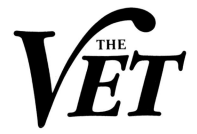

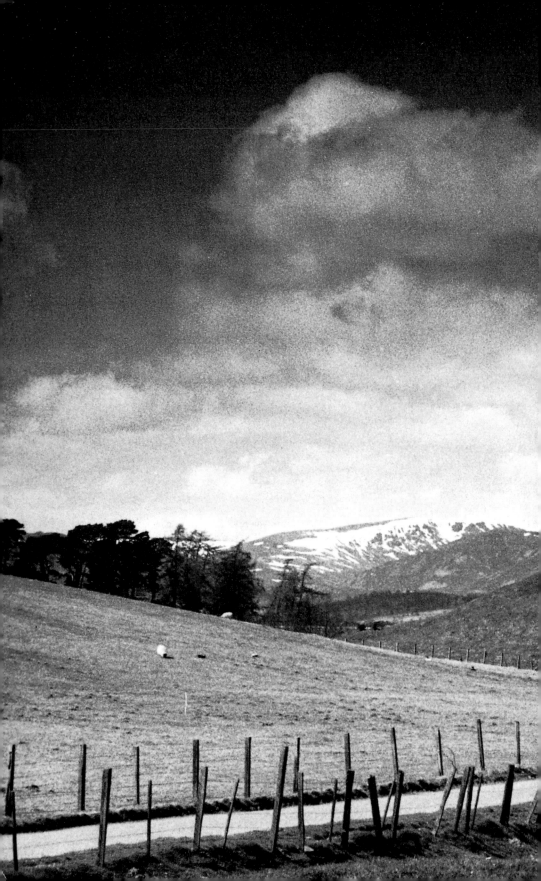

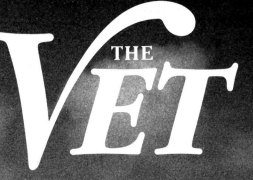

THE VET

Beyond the surgery door

GEORGE RAFFERTY
&
JEREMY MILLS

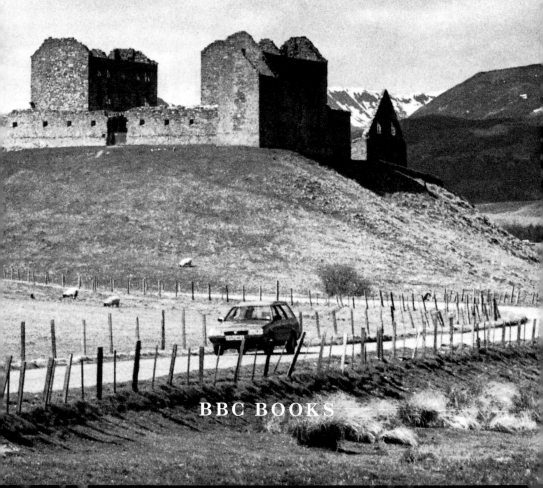

BBC BOOKS

© George Rafferty and Jeremy Mills 1989

Reprinted 1989 (twice)

Published by BBC Books
a division of BBC Enterprises Limited
Woodlands, 80 Wood Lane, London W12 OTT

ISBN 0 563 20798 1

Set in 11 on 13 Old Style by Butler & Tanner Ltd
Cover printed by Belmont
Printed and bound in Great Britain by Butler & Tanner Ltd,
Frome and London
Jacket printed by Belmont Press, Northampton

Contents

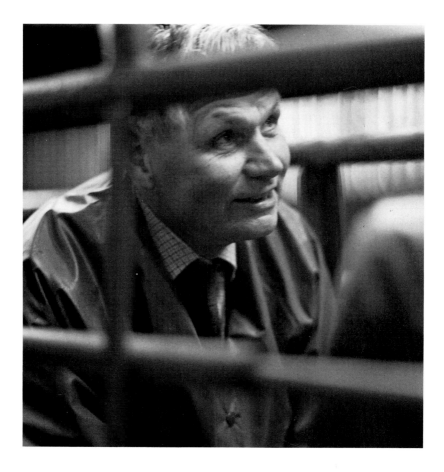

FOREWORD

IN THE SUMMER of 1988 Paul Hamann, a BBC television executive whom I'd known for a few years, introduced me to one of his producers, Jeremy Mills. They persuaded me to let Jeremy film me and the other members of my veterinary practice in Grantown-on-Spey, as we went about our daily work. Little did Jane, Willie, Neil and I know what we were letting ourselves in for. During the ensuing year Jeremy and his team (Lisa Perkins, Alex Hansen, Martyn Clift, James Moss and Pat O'Shea) followed us around the Highlands of Scotland, getting under our feet and in Jane's kitchen, in order to build up a picture of us and the community we serve.

At the same time Jeremy and I started to jot down the odd thing here and there which happened to us, our friends and the animals we treated, to help keep a record of my thoughts and the daily goings on. This book is a combination of those random jottings and some of the countless memories, good and bad, of my lifetime spent as a veterinary surgeon. It's not intended to be a comprehensive diary but merely an impression of some of the high and low points of our year.

I haven't pulled any punches because I didn't want to create too romantic an idea of our lives. Some of our work can be physically and emotionally difficult, but mostly it gives us a great deal of pleasure. I hope that reading this diary will let you share the joy of successful times and the sadness of others. If you're left with nothing but an impression of the best group of people I could ever dream of working with, and the beautiful country-side which surrounds us in this part of north-east Scotland, then I'll be happy.

GEORGE RAFFERTY
AUGUST 1989

WEDNESDAY 3 AUGUST

I T'S PULLING BACK, BOYS! I remember exclaiming. To my great surprise the calf lying inside the cow responded to my touch on its foreleg as I felt around inside the womb. The signs of life lifted my spirits and injected me with new enthusiasm.

The phone call from Willie Grant had come just after six o'clock that morning. He'd told me that he was having problems calving one of his young cows. His description of the way the calf was lying had meant that I'd driven the 20 miles to the farm at Ballantruan in the expectation of finding a dead calf, and with the prospect of hours of hard work ahead of me to get the body out and save the cow.

Willie had said that the calf was stuck in the breech position, where only the calf's tail is coming out. One of our commonest problems is that the cow has often been calving for much longer than the farmer realises. By the time help arrives the poor animal is exhausted and has given up pushing, so the calf dies. It can be very frustrating, especially when we go to a case which we could have saved if only we'd been there a bit earlier.

I'd been taken into the gloom of the ramshackle barn by Willie and his twenty-year-old nephew, young John. It's difficult to think of him as anything but 'young', knowing him as I have before he was even a twinkle in his father's eye. The black-and-white cross-bred Hereford cow was standing still on the cobbled floor, tied up by her head in one of the stalls. I could see straight away that it wasn't a breech presentation at all, but it *was* coming out backwards. There were two white hooves sticking out from the cow's rear end and I knew that if I was quick I'd be in with a chance of saving it.

A rapid examination inside the cow confirmed that it was alive and lying in the correct position to be born. It's not until you feel inside that you know for sure that the calf isn't twisted, or bent double. In this case the calf had simply got stuck because of its size, and the cow had given up. We still needed to get it out as quickly as possible though, because when calves come out backwards if you're not very careful they can drown in the fluid inside the womb. I told young John to get the calving machine from my car.

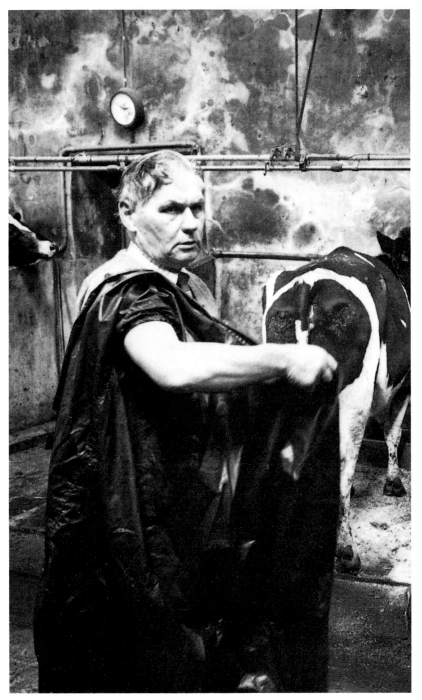

Putting on my calving gown.

'I don't know if it's us getting old or the calves getting bigger, Willie, that we need a machine to calve them.' I wondered how many times over the last third of a century Willie and I had stood in similar positions at all times of the day and night. As far as I can remember he's always worn the same flat cap, pulled down tight over his bald head. It's hard to imagine him anywhere else but in the fields or here in a barn. He'd look out of place in a town, with his big, shovel-like hands, strong, stocky body and weatherbeaten face. All the best farmers almost become part of their farms – a bit like a dry-stone wall in a field, eroded by years of exposure to the elements, yet still performing the task it was designed to do as solidly as the day it was built. I suppose Willie will be getting on a bit now, but then that's true of many of my clients these days. No doubt they would remind me that I also said cheerio to my sixtieth birthday a while ago. The farmers in Strathspey are a pretty hardy bunch, solid in build and character, and I always feel privileged to work alongside them.

'Aye, vet, I tried to pull it oot but it just wouldnae come.' I looked at Willie as he spoke in his strong Highland accent. If the power in his thick arms wasn't enough to pull the calf into the world, I knew that even the machine would have its work cut out.

Young John, who's a younger version of his uncle, returned with the calving machine and a grin. 'You must have come into money, George; this machine's brand new. I hope it doesn't mean you'll be putting your fees up!'

The calving machine is a long metal bar with notches in it. One end has a T-piece across it which I told Willie to brace against the cow's backside. I got John to put his foot on the other end to keep it firmly in place on the cobbles. I tied one end of a rope around the calf's legs and the other on to the moving part of the machine. This is a block which has a ratchet mechanism operated by a handle. Every time you move the handle to and fro, the block moves along another notch, farther away from the cow, pulling the calf out inch by inch.

IN THE OLD days we didn't have anything but our own strength to calve a cow. Whenever you turned up at a farm there would be four or five strapping men to help with the birth. We'd simply tie a rope around the calf and pull. When I had to go to a calving case in the middle of the night I used to be quite annoyed if there weren't three or four men there ready to help. If it was just a farmer on his own he would rush around the nearby farms and get his neighbours out. It was always a real social occasion, great camaraderie, a bit like a rugby team – and I'm sure that sometimes we must have looked like a rugby team as well, all pulling on the ropes tied to the calf, and pushing the cow. If it was a really big calf and we didn't have enough muscle power with the men that were there, we'd send into the farmhouse and get the farmer's wife and daughter out. And they'd come out in their flannelette nightgowns to help pull. Very often an extra woman on the ropes was enough to get the calf out.

There have been other times when I've been driven to more drastic measures. I remember one calving case at the Slochd which is on the main A9 on the way to Inverness. I was calving a heifer, a young cow, with a big calf inside her. It was just the farmer, me and his wife and we got kind of stuck with the calf halfway out. I thought, heck, what can I do. So I ran out on to the A9 road and stopped the first vehicle that came along. It happened to be the AA man.

I explained that there was an emergency with a cow and asked if he'd mind coming in to help us. I thought he might have asked if I was an AA member, but he didn't and readily offered his services. Apart from shouting orders at him during the operation I didn't really give him a second glance until after we'd calved the cow. Then I turned to thank him and compliment him on doing a good job. As soon as I looked at him properly I recognised him as a farmer's son from the other side of the practice. He was really quite amused at the whole affair. He said that he'd joined the AA to get away from farming, and here he was doing exactly what he'd been brought up to do all his life. He was obviously destined to be haunted by farming. I haven't had to resort to such desperate measures since the calving machine was introduced about fifteen years ago.

After a calving we'd all go into the house and the wife would make tea, and there was usually a dram (which, for all you readers south of the border, I'd better explain, is a tot of whisky). If it was during the night no one was in a hurry to get home and we'd sit about chatting. I'd really enjoy those times. There's nothing as pleasurable as a dram of whisky you've earned. Sometimes it would take half an hour to calve the cow and another couple of hours having tea and chatting, but it wasn't wasted time as it would have been during the day – I'd only be sleeping otherwise.

THE RHYTHMIC CLICK of the ratchet sounded loud in Willie's small barn. It was doing its job well. Gradually more and more of the matted fur of the black-and-white calf was appearing. It's not only the change in manpower which has encouraged the use of the machine over the last few years. Society has forced agriculture into producing higher yields from all areas of farming, including livestock. We now cross our cows with continental bulls and they produce calves which are up to twenty-five per cent bigger than the ones when I started out in practice over forty years ago. Some of the big continental calves can weigh over a hundredweight. This means that we're bound to have more problems with calves literally getting stuck. I remember one of the local farmers' daughters, Mary Anne Nicolson, saying to me once when we were hard at work in the depths of the night calving one such cross-bred calf, 'George, when I get married I'm looking for a man with a small head and a small pelvis.'

Looking at the strain that poor cow was under at that moment I thought Mary Anne was very wise! At least with the machine the cow is braced so that there's more traction and less of a drag across the barn, and her suffering is limited to a few minutes rather than hours.

The calf's legs came out without too much problem, then the body. But it stuck again as the front quarters presented themselves. 'Push, lassie, push.' I could feel drops of sweat running into my eyes as the effort needed to operate the handle became greater.

Then all of a sudden the front quarters of the calf appeared, and I knew that the worst was over. Winded by the effort I gasped to young John to operate the handle while I supported the calf's body as it came out. Before John could get to the handle the calf had literally slipped out, and I just managed to catch it before it hit the hard cobbled floor.

This was the point where speed was essential. 'Take her leg, John, and swing when I say.' John hardly needed my prompting; he must have been involved in enough of these situations to know by now what to do. We swung the calf by its hind legs a few times. It's like doctors giving a baby a smack on the bottom: it makes them react and hopefully cough up anything in their throats before there's a danger of them choking on it. There's nothing more annoying and distressing than seeing a calf which is technically alive – you can see the heart beating – but it can't take a breath because it's all choked with fluid from the womb and then it dies in your hands.

'Quick, boys, over the door with it.' We carried the calf, covered in blood and afterbirth, to the stable door. It was one of those doors with two sections, top and bottom, and we lifted the body across the closed bottom section.

'It's breathing, George,' There was no disguising the delight on Willie's face as he said this.

I had no hesitation in joining in his pleasure. 'Aye that fair makes my day too, Willie, to get a live calf out.' And it does. All the hard work was worth it.

I was puffing and panting, though, from the effort. Young John was grinning all over his face. 'The vet's worn out!' He couldn't resist a dig.

After a few deep lungfuls of crisp air, I recovered enough to confirm that it was a girl. As we cleaned the mouth out the calf gave a cough and a shake of its head as though to ask what all the fuss was about.

We lifted the calf off the door and on to the floor. Willie put a piece of straw up its nose to make it sneeze and help clear all the nasal passages. I'm sure my more modern colleagues would laugh at some of the old fashioned ways in these parts but as far as I'm concerned they seem to work as well as any of the new methods, so why stop them just for the sake of so-called progress.

'What's this, George?' Willie was pointing to a small black lump on the calf's back.

I took a look. 'I haven't seen that for years, Willie. It's a sort of birth-mark. We'll leave it for a few weeks, then I'll come and cut it out.'

I examined the cow who had stood quietly throughout the birth, although she'd had a lot of pulling about. Remarkably, she was fine. Animals are a lot tougher than humans. If a woman had been through what that cow had she'd be confined to bed for days to recover. But as soon as I'd given her a shot of penicillin to stop any infection, young John released the head chain and she moved across to her calf and started licking it. Cows are really very simple creatures; they don't have complex feelings like, say, dogs do. They care about food, they understand pain, but above all they have strong instincts to care for their young. They always look proud when they see the calf for the first time, and they like to show off their new-born offspring. These instincts can be so strong that they turn aggressive towards anyone or anything they think is threatening their calf. One farmer not so long ago got charged, knocked down and had his collar-bone broken. It really made quite a mess of him. Sometimes a cow will go off her head after calving and even attack her own calf and really throw it about. So we've got to watch them, and I try to make a rule to stand between them and the door ready for a quick getaway if necessary.

IN TODAY'S CASE, though, the cow showed no interest in us. She was too concerned about her youngster to waste any of the energy she had left on even giving us another thought. Her rough tongue seemed to lick new life into the lump of matted hair. The licking and nudging from a good mother stimulates the calf. It makes it aware that it's in the big bad world and has to look after itself, get up on its feet and suck. At first it made a few tentative attempts to lever itself up on its front legs. Then its hind legs were given a work-out, and before too long the calf was trying to stand and suckle. All that from something which only an hour or so earlier everyone had thought to be dead.

The sooner the calf sucks the better, because the first milk in the udder, the colostrum, is full of antibodies and vitamins. When the calf is just a few hours old it's able to absorb these from its mother's milk. That gives it resistance to all sorts of disease, and ultimately helps it grow better.

'That's a good morning's work, Willie. You'll deserve a wee dram tonight!' I smiled with full knowledge that we'd shared a dram or two of whisky on these occasions over the years.

'Aye, George, and no doubt you'll have one yourself to wet the baby's head!' Willie had that sort of twinkle in his eye which comes from knowing me too well!

I ALWAYS GET a great feeling coming away from a calving case when I've had to do a bit of hard work and at the end of it the result is good. The farmer's happy, the calf's alive, and it makes all the humdrum everyday work of the practice worthwhile. It's not only the financial side of things, although I suppose a female calf like that would be worth around £200 to the farmer, but the feeling that if I hadn't been there it wouldn't have been born alive. I'm lucky that I can say that most of my clients are also my friends, so I also get pleasure from knowing that it's a small help towards their business.

AS I WAS driving away from Ballantruan I couldn't help smiling as I remembered a story often told about the previous tenant, Elsie MacArthur. She'd been there for many years as had her father before her, and there was a man who worked for her called Jock. To all outward appearances Jock was the worker and Elsie was the farmer, all very right and proper. Jock slept in the bothy (the accommodation for single farm hands) and he fed in the kitchen, and as far as anyone knew that was it.

One night there were some army manoeuvres going on in Avonside nearby and there had been lorries going up and down the road all through the night. The next day Jock met a neighbouring farmer, Donald. They'd been discussing all the commotion during the night and Jock said to Donald, 'I just turned over to Elsie and said, "You would think it was the invasion all over again."' Of course nothing was said but like everything up here it was soon all around the district that there was more to their relationship than people had previously thought. I suppose that sort of news travels fast in any small community.

REMEMBERING THAT STORY about Jock and Elsie increased my good humour, and I really enjoyed the drive back to Grantown. So much so that I even noticed the scenery. It usually takes a visitor to point out the beauty of the area, with the Cairngorms rising above the River Spey. However, this morning, at a time when most visitors hadn't even thought of starting on their bacon and eggs, with the sun out in a clear blue August sky and the roads to myself, it would have been difficult not to appreciate how lucky I am to be living in this part of the world. I often think that Great Britain is the best country in the world, and we live in the best part of that country. It's strange that after all these years and I suppose thousands of births I still get the same sense of achievement now that I did forty years ago when I went to my first calving case.

JUST AFTER I qualified in 1948 I went to work in Hereford with a chap called Barker who had a great reputation as a cattle vet. It wasn't long before I was sent out to my first solo calving case. Calving gowns had just started to be used in the profession to protect the animal and the vet, but Mr Barker didn't believe in using them. 'Waste of money, old boy!' he used to say – and he supplied his people with pyjama jackets instead.

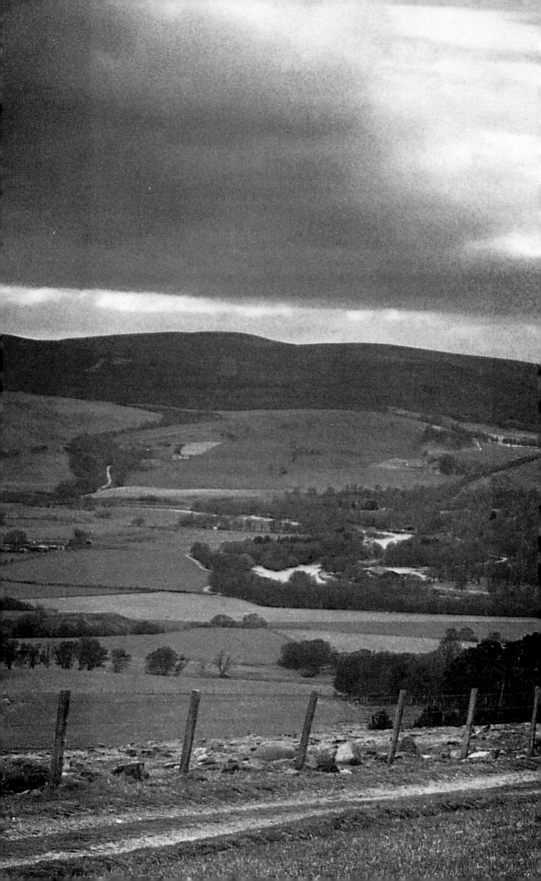

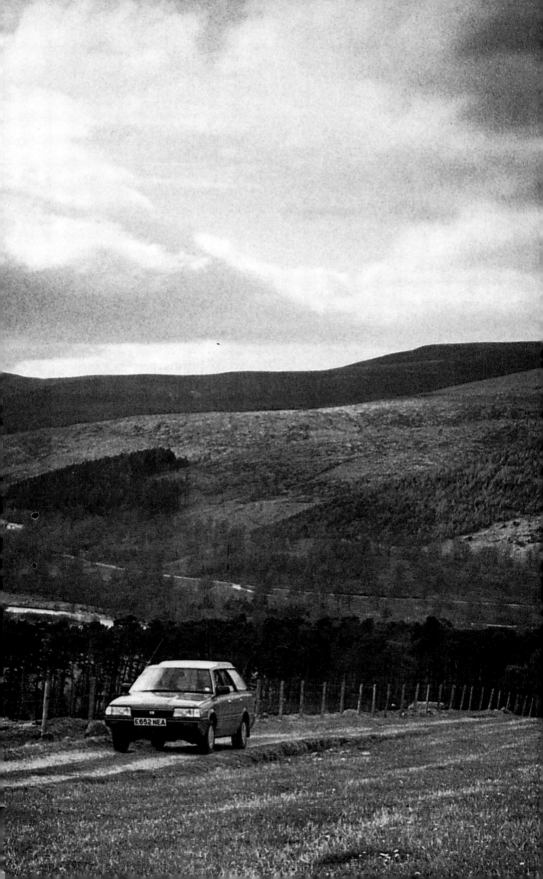

When I first saw him in his uniform I realised that I'd joined the wrong profession if I wanted to look elegant. He was a very large man and he certainly looked quite a sight in his old pyjama top which had seen more use than was decent. Unfortunately the jackets only covered the top half of the body, although mine went down to my knees. A pair of oilskin trousers were essential to complete the outfit. I hadn't been able to buy any at that point, and my only legwear was a new pair of expensive cavalry twill trousers, which cost quite a lot in those days. I really was very proud of them.

The calving case was a heifer with a very large calf inside her. I had four or five men helping me, and bottle of linseed oil. This was my boss's magic touch. He insisted on its use to lubricate the vagina, and make the birth canal slippery so that the calf would ease out with no problem.

I got down to business with the linseed oil well in attendance and had quite a job getting the calf away from the heifer. Eventually after a struggle the calf was born safely and with no real problems. Except, that is, for my smart new trousers. I'd been so intent on the job that I hadn't noticed what a mess I'd been getting into. I stood up and removed the pyjama jacket to discover that the cavalry twills which, just moments earlier, had been my pride and joy were now a nasty slippery sticky mess.

I was in digs with no facilities for washing, and there were no launderettes those days, so, sad to say, they were unredeemable and thrown away after a single wearing. It was a hard way to learn that the right clothes for the job are essential.

The boss was a very big man and like most professional men a bit of an actor and very conscious of his image. He used to drive a big new car, a Ford V8. In 1948 just after the war there weren't many about, so this guaranteed that he was always noticed. That and his dress sense. He used to wear a blue serge suit and a polka dot bow tie. When he went to see a sick animal he would get out of the car, and stand and look the animal over. Then he'd get out his tobacco and his cigarette paper and roll his own cigarettes – he never bought ready made ones. All the time he rolled the cigarette he'd be talking to the farmer, asking questions about the animal and studying it. That made a tremendous impression on me and ever since I've always spent a few moments standing looking at the animal and asking plenty of questions before doing anything. The only difference is that I don't smoke! When you're newly qualified you're inclined to go rushing in, stethoscope and thermometer in hand, taking the animal's temperature and pulse and listening to its chest. Sometimes doing that you miss an awful lot. I've been grateful to him ever since.

BACK HOME I opened the day's post which had arrived while I'd been out on the call. Some results of blood tests, a few bills and even the odd payment cheque. Then a shortish, round man, with curly black hair going grey at the sides and bald in the middle, and with his glasses perpetually perched on the end of his nose, appeared around the kitchen door. Willie Hollick has been an assistant with me for about sixteen years now and is as much a part of the household as we are ourselves. We consulted the day's page in the diary and I decided who was to see which cases. Willie bustled about getting the drugs ready and set off on his calls. During the day most of our work is on the farms, unless there's an emergency with a small animal in which case one of us will rush back to the surgery.

I'm an old fashioned veterinary surgeon. The practice is run from the house. It's a bit like farming where the wife is very much involved in the business. Jane is more than involved, she's vital to the whole operation. Everything is here. The kitchen is office, reception, rest room, restaurant, recovery room and lots more. On one side of the kitchen is the waiting room and surgery, on the other a storeroom-cum-dispensary, and beyond that the rest of the house.

Because of all this there's one thing a veterinary surgeon needs, and that's an understanding wife. Even the simple domestic chores are worse than most people would put up with. Very often your clothes get into a bit of a mess, especially on a calving case. Quite often the blood discharged gets in under the calving gown and it's not uncommon to have to change shirts a few times a day when we're busy. Jane can gauge how many calving cases we're doing just by the number of shirts she has to wash. The moment I walked in the door and she saw the state of my shirt, she'd got a clean one ready for me and the dirty one was away to be washed. She uses the old fashioned way of getting rid of stains, by laying the clothes out on the grass and letting the sun bleach them.

Even though each day is different we've got a routine going. The calls start coming in after half past seven, and they all go down in the diary. I decide which of us does which call and in what order. From then on Jane takes over and when the new calls come in she decides whether they are emergencies or can wait until one of us gets back. She always knows where we are and how to get hold of us if she needs to. After all these years she has a pretty good idea of priorities.

I was in the main street in Grantown once on my way to an emergency case, when a farmer came up to me and started in: 'I've got this old cow which has—' Before he could continue I cut him off: 'I've no time now. I'm in a hell of a rush!'

Without showing any irritation at my abrupt interruption he replied, 'Aye well, don't worry, Vet, I'll go down and see your wifee. She knows as much as you do about cows!' And you know he was probably right. The farmers say that she often gives better advice over the phone than I do! Jane is a vital member of the team – as well as being my sleeping partner she's also a working partner. I often refer to her as the Managing Director, because she really does organise the practice. She stays at the house all day keeping the phone by her for any calls. She is the brains of the business, and without her the whole thing would go to pot. The other weekend she went off for a couple of days to see the family down in Lanarkshire and we were running around like a load of chickens with our heads cut off! Mind you, she's a devil for taking holidays: she goes away for two weekends a year to see the grandchildren. I always make a point of telling her how much we've missed her, so that she won't go off too often.

I don't think there's anything better for a woman than to know that she's needed; it makes her content with her lot even though her lot might be hard. And Jane's lot is certainly tougher than most women I know. But there's nothing like plenty of hard work to keep a woman happy, and she's certainly got lots of that!

WITH THE LARGE area we cover in the practice people often ask me why we don't carry any of the new communication equipment. But I can't be doing with all this new technology; it's mostly a waste of time and money as far as I'm concerned. I always say that as soon as they invent a computer which wakes you up with a nudge in the middle of the night and says, 'You forgot to do so and so,' then I'll buy one. Until that time I'm quite happy with one that keeps me warm as well! Besides, we have a simple way of keeping in touch with what's going on. At any time of the day

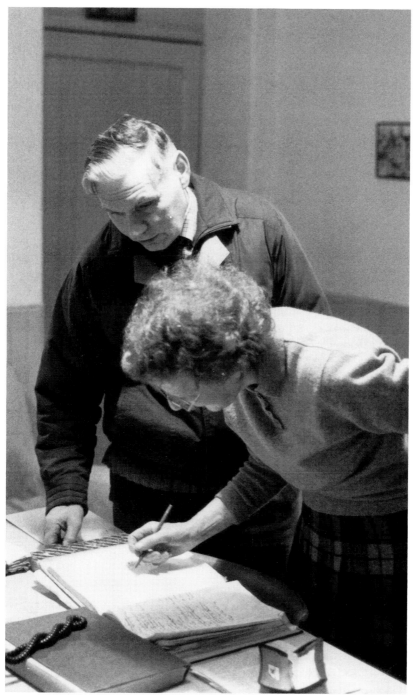

Arranging the day's duties with Jane before setting off on the rounds.

Jane can look at the diary and see where we should be, then she can phone the farm and they pass on the message. Mind you, this system can have its disadvantages – Jane knows by now how long each job should take, which is great from the work point of view, but it does mean that staying sitting in someone's kitchen having a dram can be a bit dangerous! It doesn't take Jane long to work out that we're behind schedule and she has a pretty good idea of where the extra time's gone! I suppose that with a bleeper we could always claim that it was out of range or something.

THINKING ABOUT NEW technology always takes me back to our early days in Grantown in the 1950s when there were very few telephones. Without the aid of any of this new stuff we evolved a system of keeping in touch when I was out on calls. I think it was much more interesting than anything technology has to offer.

The local policeman, Mackay, lived on a strategic corner of the road between Glenlivet and Grantown and when a farmer in the area wanted to get in touch with me Jane would phone up and get Mackay to put out a flag. The same system of communication was used for the doctor, so the code we developed was a white flag for the vet and a red one for the doctor – I'm sure there was no significance in the choice of colours! It all seemed to work very well. I would see the flag, stop and get my instructions. It eventually spread in use so that anyone wanting to get hold of me would put something white out to attract my attention. I would go batting around a corner, see something white, and know to call in. A list of the items put into service for this purpose might make a few people blush – some of them were certainly very arresting!

Mackay told me a story about one farmer who rang to get him to put the flag out for me. His name was Alan and he had a very bad stutter. He phoned one day and said, 'C-C-C-C-Can you l-l-l-leave a m-m-m-m-message for the v-v-v-et.'

'Yes, Alan, of course,' said Mackay.

There was a pause at the other end, and then Alan's puzzled voice came back down the line. 'H-H-H-How did y-y-y-y-y-you know it it w-w-w-was me?'

THE REST OF today was fairly ordinary. A call to Tomintoul, then down to a couple of farms along the River Spey to do some routine vaccinations of cattle. Then a house call on a dog which

I seem to get called to every few weeks. I've a feeling the wifee just wants a bit of company, more than really thinking there's anything wrong with the dog, but then in a small community like ours that sort of thing's all part of the job, I suppose. I always say that we're jacks of all trades – what the plumber or the doctor can't sort out we have to cope with.

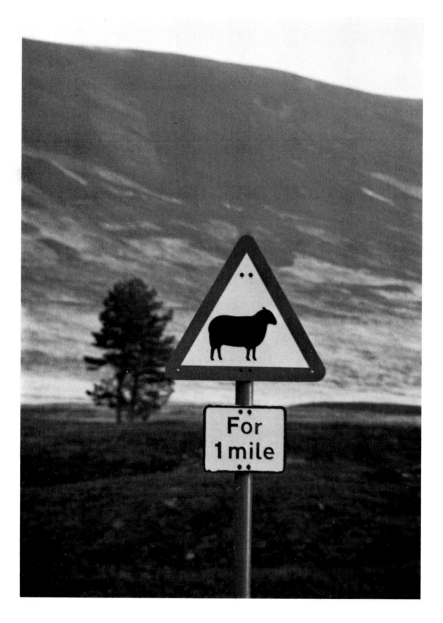

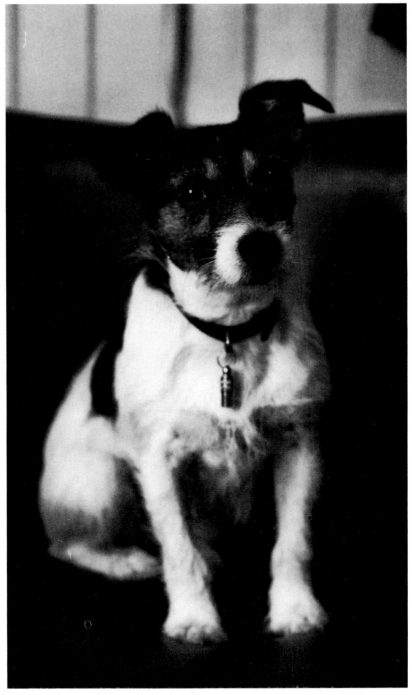

Corrie

MONDAY 8 AUGUST

I T W A S S I X o'clock this evening when I turned into our road. Evening surgery starts at half past six, but people often get there early. As I drove down the road I looked to see if any cars were parked outside. Whenever there are, I know that it might still be some time before I get anything to eat – it's no use telling a dog which needs stitches in a wound that you'll see to it as soon as you've had your tea!

Tonight there were several cars already parked and I must admit my heart sank for a moment. But I knew that a familiar sight would be waiting for me as I pulled into the drive – Corrie, my Jack Russell. She usually hears the car coming down the road and leaps up on to the back of my armchair to look out of the kitchen window, her tail wagging excitedly. This never fails to lift my spirits even after a hard day. As I got out of the car she bounded down from the chair and rushed to the door, ready to give me an enthusiastic greeting.

THE WAITING ROOM was full of dogs tonight, all trying to have their say. It sounded a bit like the canine equivalent of the United Nations, all different breeds talking away to each other and getting a wee bit agitated. It's quite usual to find that once an animal has been into the surgery it seems to recognise the smell of antiseptic or something. If its previous experience was an unpleasant one, it tends not to be too happy about paying us a return visit!

With the number of people waiting there was nothing for it but to get stuck in and sort out the ones making the most noise first. When I put on my white coat all thoughts of food disappeared.

MRS WILLMOT CARRIED a small black-and-white Jack Russell bitch into the surgery, while her two daughters followed with a cardboard box. I lifted the box on to the examination table and saw two tiny pups inside. They'd come to get their dew claws removed – a small operation, but essential for their health.

The bitch, with her tongue hanging out and panting away, strained to see into the box and check that her youngsters were still safe. If you want to see maternal instincts at their most potent and basic you only have to watch animals with their offspring: this dog was desperate to check that her pups were not being harmed in any way. For such a small dog she was proving to be difficult to restrain.

By now both the pups in their makeshift carrier had started to yelp, which in turn started the mother off again. The high-pitched noise was getting unbearable.

'I'll give her one of the pups to lick while we deal with the other.' I said, and, sure enough, as soon as I handed over one of the tiny bundles the noise stopped and there was a welcome moment of quiet in the confined space of the surgery.

As the noise stopped, Willie came in, hair tousled, glasses on the end of his nose again, and a big grin for everyone in the room. I'd no need to ask how his afternoon had gone. Jane told me that he'd been out to a calving case, and, like me, his mood is always a dead giveaway as to whether he's been successful or not. Tonight the grin and bounce in his step told me that straight away. I called him over to give me a hand.

'Get your white coat on, Willie, and we'll get these two wee pups sorted out. Have you washed your hands?'

'Och yes, I'm all ready.'

It's often struck me that for an Englishman Willie has picked up more of the mannerisms of a Scotsman than many of the locals! He's been an assistant with me for sixteen years now, and even now I sometimes have to remind myself that he's not the young novice that I took on all those years ago, but an experienced and well respected vet.

As he bent over the box to pick up our first patient, Willie's glasses slid even further down his nose. The wee pup, only a few days old, was small enough to fit comfortably into the palm of his hand. Taking the surgical scissors I cut the first dew claw off, chatting to Mrs Willmot the while.

'How's your mother, Mrs Willmot?'

'Oh not too bad now, Mr Rafferty. She's able to walk again now, but she has problems if she does too much.'

'Well you'll have to make sure she takes it easy – tell her from me that she'll have to give the Grantown marathon a miss this year. I might stand a chance of winning it then!'

Mrs Willmot laughed. I suppose in a way I enjoy talking to the people as much as I do treating the animals. In forty-odd years of practice I must have done this particular job hundreds of times. One of the great joys about being as long in the tooth as me is that you can do the job and chat away at the same time. After all, keeping the owners happy and relaxed helps to keep the pets calm as well. An owner who's all twitchy will soon make the animal nervous. Something you notice about newly qualified vets is the amount of concentration they need to do even these simple jobs.

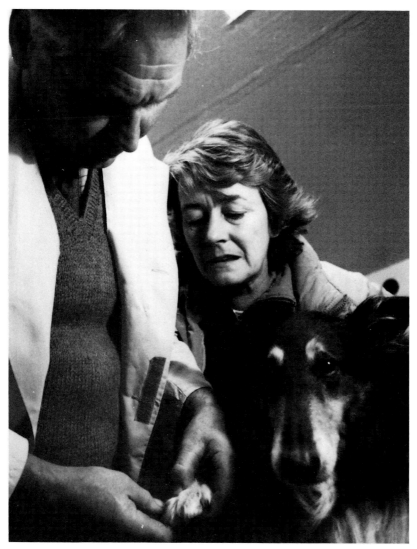

The initial examination – an anxious moment for every owner.

'Hang on, I'll turn the pup around so you can get at that one more easily,' said Willie. It whimpered slightly as he moved it around.

Hearing its distress, Mrs Willmot cleared her throat and reluctantly, almost defensively, asked, 'I'm never sure whether this is really necessary for the dog's health. Do you think it is, Mr Rafferty?'

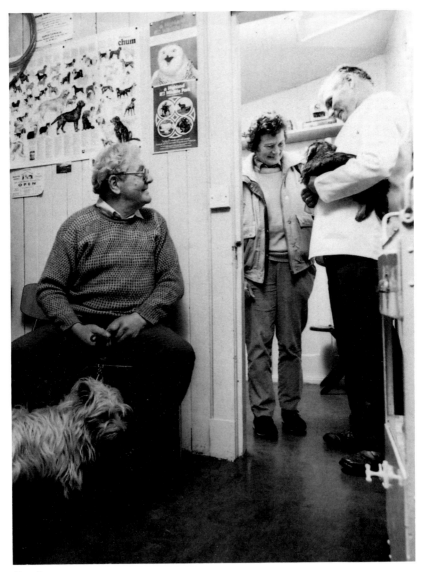

Evening surgery

'Oh yes, definitely.' I explained that the dew claws are small fingers really that grow halfway up the leg and quite often get caught when the dogs scrabble around in rough bracken and heather. Then they get torn, and they can cause all kinds of problems.

Morag, one of Mrs Willmot's daughters who'd been watching what we'd been doing with great concentration, piped up, 'Why do they have them then?'

I explained that in the past, before people had them as pets, before they were given tinned food to eat, the dogs had to fend for themselves and they used their claws for fighting. So they really don't need them any more. If we leave them, they often have to have them removed when they're adult dogs, but then it becomes a small operation with an anaesthetic and so on. At this age they hardly feel anything because the nerves aren't properly formed. It's more like having one of your toenails cut.

My explanation seemed to satisfy the girl, who returned to watching the work intently.

Next we had to dock the tail. Willie turned the puppy so that I could get at it with the scissors. I have to admit that this is a purely cosmetic operation. The Jack Russell naturally has a long tail and the fashion is to have them short. I have to admit that I don't like doing it, but I'd rather perform the operation myself than have the owners do it at home, on the kitchen table – perhaps with disastrous results. In reality it's one of the practices which will continue as long as the Kennel Club keeps tail cropping as one of the requirements for some breeds. If they dropped it then the practice would probably die out.

'What do you think, Willie? Is that the right length?'

'Aye, that looks about right, maybe just leave a wee bit more black.'

'Just pinch the tail as I cut it then, Willie.' We don't use an anaesthetic for this; pinching the tail is enough to deaden any sensation. A snip with the scissors and it was off. Then I cauterised it to make sure it didn't bleed.

'There you are, Mrs Willmot. It didn't seem to mind that too much. Right, we'll swop them over now and do the other one. Here you are, wee dog, here's your baby.'

The mother took the young pup and licked it vigorously as we started on the second one. Through the surgery door I could hear the other dogs getting restless again, but the second pup didn't take long to do and they were soon ready to leave.

'Who's next, please?' I asked the full waiting room.

'I think it's me, Mr Rafferty.'

'Where's your animal, Mrs Money?'

'Outside in the drive.'

In this job you never know what sort of animal you're going to be treating next. Why hadn't Mrs Money brought her animal in? My mind started to run through all the possibilities, but as soon as I walked outside I could see why she had left it there. It was a donkey that stood patiently waiting behind my car.

'She's got an abscess here at the top of her foreleg.' Mrs Money pointed carefully.

'I'm glad it's not on her hind leg, Mrs Money!' I replied, feelingly, remembering the odd occasion when my attentions had been awarded with a good kick.

I examined the donkey and sure enough it had an abscess which would need an injection of antibiotics to get rid of the infection.

I've known Mrs Money for years. She's a real animal person – and a generous one too. I often find that she's paid for someone else to bring their sick animal to us. We don't get cruelty to animals in this part of the world; the worst sort of case we come across might be someone with a cat needing spaying or neutering who can't afford to have it done. Then someone like Mrs Money will usually pay. Either that or we don't get any money.

'I'll need to get the injection and a razor to shave her, Mrs Money.'

Running back through the crowded waiting room I apologised for keeping everyone waiting. In the surgery Willie was dealing with a small brown hamster which wasn't eating, brought in by a small boy who looked as though he ate a bit too much himself. It was hard to keep a straight face as I overheard part of the conversation.

'Why do you think he *should* eat chocolate?' asked Willie in a voice thick with forced patience.

'Well, it's what I like,' said the boy, implying that the answer was obvious. Unfortunately I missed the rest of the conversation since I had collected everything I needed from the surgery drawers. No doubt Willie would soon have that particular problem sorted out.

The light was fading fast outside. Luckily it didn't take long

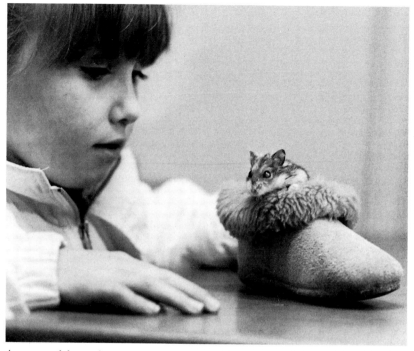

An unusual form of transport for this Russian hamster.

to shave the hair around the abscess and inject the drugs. The donkey stood pretty docile during the injection but didn't take too kindly to having some ointment rubbed into the wound, and lunged forward towards the surgery door dragging Mrs Money with it, nearly knocking over an old lady with a Pekinese dog. Luckily before any damage could be caused the donkey decided it'd had enough and let Mrs Money lead it back up the drive.

The surgery carried on in similar fashion until just before eight o'clock. Eventually the last owner departed, having been reassured that her dog was well. Sometimes I wonder if some of the owners project their own hypochondria on to their pets.

I turned out the lights in the waiting room. In the surgery Willie had already given an anaesthetic to a small black-and-white dog with a broken leg.

'It's been in before, hasn't it, Willie?'

'Aye, it came in about a year ago. It belongs to that family of gypsies who live just out of town.'

'Oh, I know. Well we'll be lucky to be paid for this job then, Willie.'

I suppose I should have a different attitude towards our payment system. It's not that we're lax about sending out bills – far from it, Jane is very efficient. She spends an hour or so every night keeping the accounts up to date. But in a place where we know everyone's business we usually have a fairly accurate picture of who can afford to pay and who can't. You'd have to be a hard-hearted kind of person to insist on cash before treatment. That would only mean that they wouldn't bring their animals in to us, and I hate to think of that happening. I'm not saying that we run any sort of charity; we most certainly don't! We're here to make money. At the end of the day, though, I can usually balance the books. Maybe one or two southerners who come up here on holiday get charged the odd few pence over if I know they can afford it, to make up for the rest. Even for them our prices are probably lower than anywhere in the country so they don't do too badly.

'Come on, wee dog. What sort is it, Willie?'

'I'm not sure. I think it's a bit of Heinz – 57 varieties.'

While we were talking we laid out sheets of old *Financial Times* on the operating table. I prefer the *Financial Times* because it's the most absorbing and the most absorbent paper. I think they must use some different kind of printing paper. It's better than using special disposable paper, because we can read this first! This being Scotland we like to keep the costs down every way possible. After all, it all has to come out of the fees we earn, so the less we spend the less we have to charge, and the more that ordinary folk can afford to come to us.

I don't like to waste money in the surgery in any way. That's why we don't have masses of stainless steel surfaces and all the latest gear. I know that some of the student vets we get are a bit taken aback when they first see the surgery and waiting room – two small rooms next to the kitchen. One student even said that it was like photographs he'd seen in books about veterinary history! It's true most of the stuff is pretty old – but why buy new stuff for the sake of it? It all does exactly what we ask of it. Any fool can spend money, but it takes a wise man to save it!

The operating and examination table is one of my favourite examples of that thriftiness. Stan Hendry, the dentist in town, was putting in one of these modern chairs in his surgery and asked me if I'd like the old one. So we got the blacksmith to put a table-top on it, and it does the job perfectly. We can move it up and down and it swivels, and it cost a fraction of the hundreds of

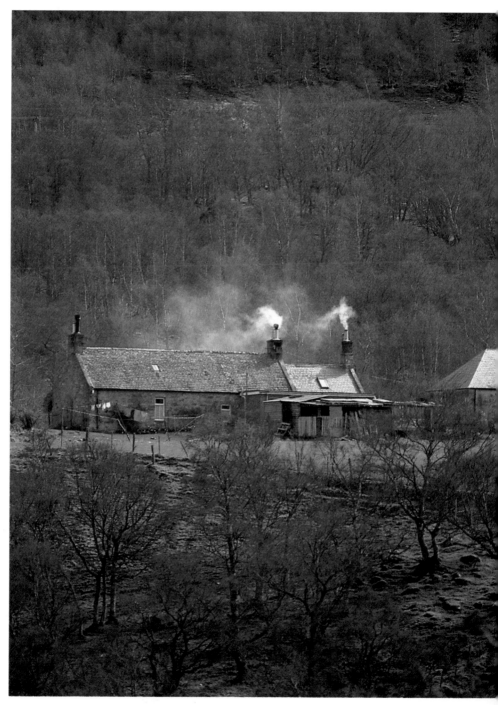
Smoke from a peat fire drifts across a remote croft.

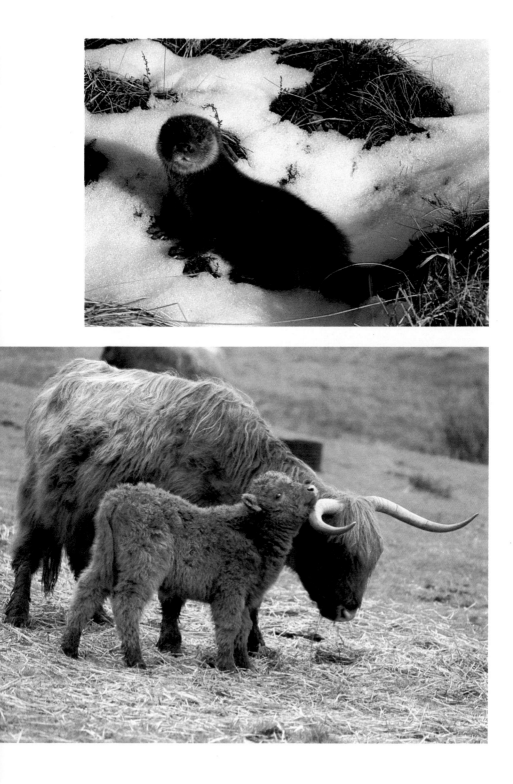

Left above   *Baby otter at the Highland Wildlife Park near Aviemore.*

Left below   *Highland cattle at the Wildlife Park.*

Right   *Canon Arthur Wheatley and his new pup BJ, daughter of Sparta.*

Below   *Willie Grant of Ballantruan.*

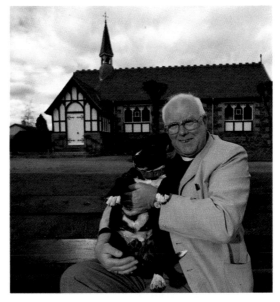

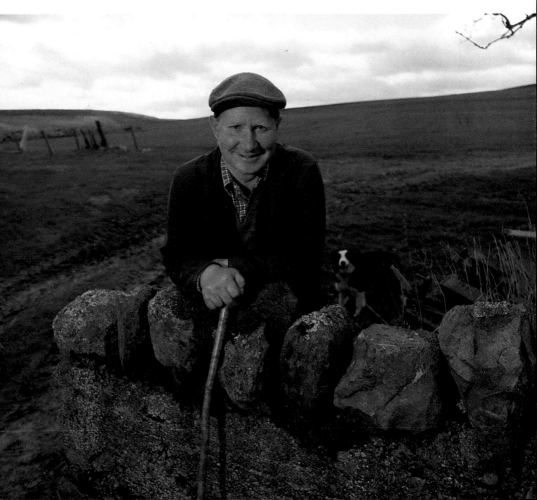

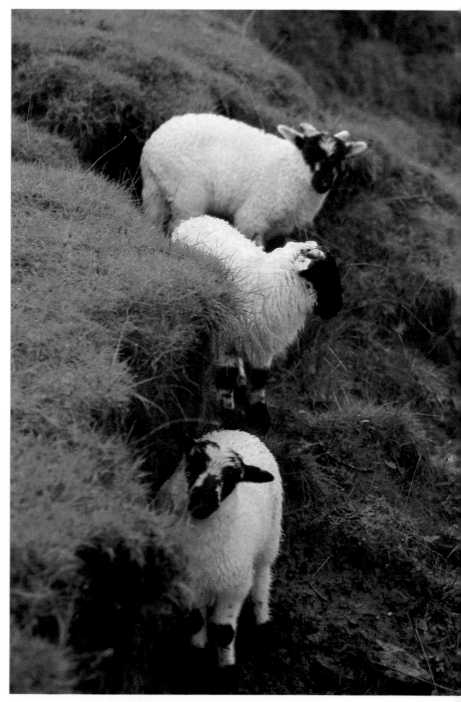

Sheep by a burn in the Highlands.

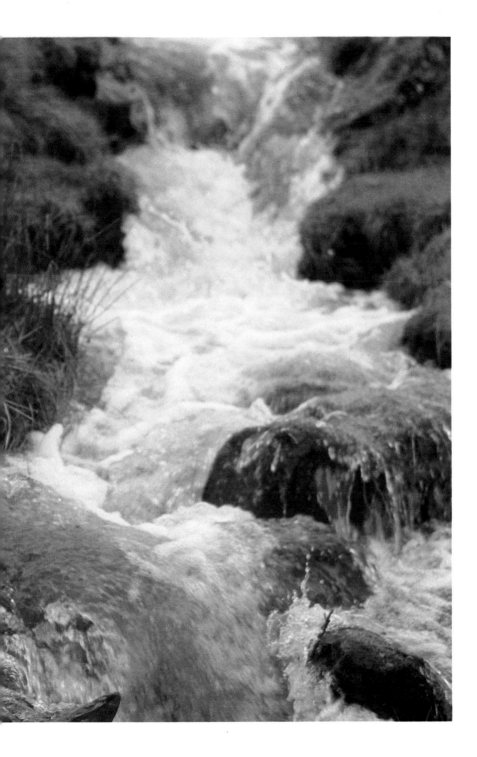

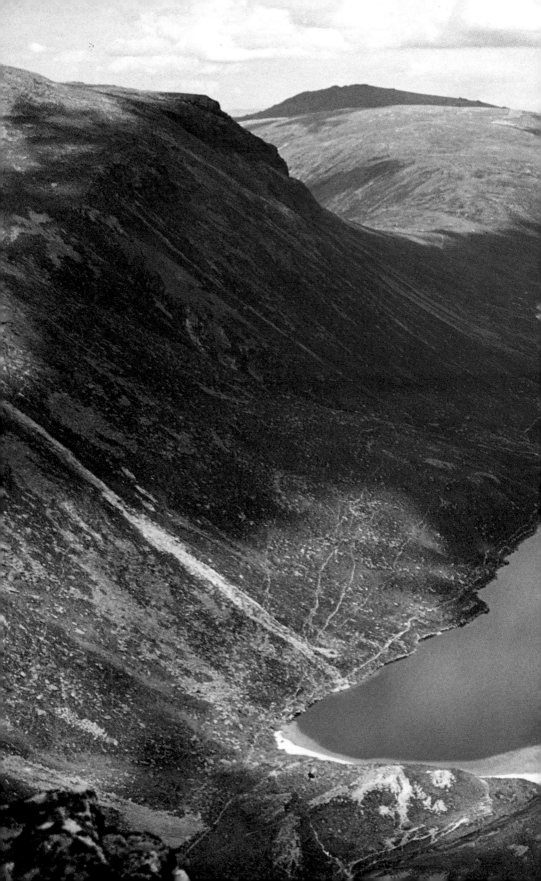

The view over Loch Avon never fails to take my breath away.

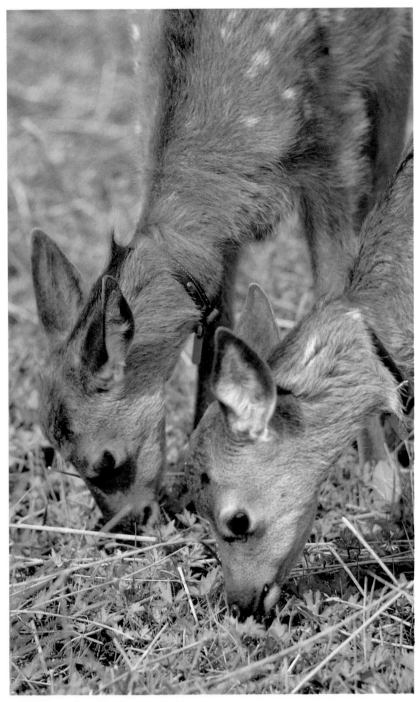

Red deer calves at the Highland Wildlife Park.

pounds a purpose-built table would have done, which wouldn't have served our needs any better.

EVERYTHING WAS READY now. The dog was out cold, and the special plastic bandage we use to set animals' broken legs was hot. It's a sort of very fine white mesh which becomes pliable in boiling water, and then sets rock solid when it cools. It does the same job as plaster of Paris, without any of the mess. You just mould it around the leg to give maximum support and immobilise it. It's great here in the surgery, but not so good out in the open, especially in the winter. You have to work very quickly before it cools in low temperatures.

It was quite an easy job, setting the leg, and the sort of operation which gives us a chance to talk and catch up on what we've both been up to during the day.

'How was Wee Dod's cow today, Willie?'

'Just fine, I don't think we'll need to go back to her unless he phones tomorrow.'

'Another satisfied customer.'

'I wouldn't go as far as that. He was having his usual moan about vets' fees!'

I couldn't help laughing. I've been going to Wee Dod's for as long as I've been in Grantown and he's always moaned about something. It's become a ritual; it doesn't mean anything.

'It was a busy surgery tonight, Willie.'

'Aye, did you see that boy with the wee hamster?'

'Well I heard you talking to him. What was that all about chocolate?'

'Well he thought that because he liked it so would his hamster!'

My thoughts about owners surfaced. 'Why the hell didn't his father sort it out?'

'I think his dad wanted him to take responsibility for his own animal, and come in and sort the problem out himself.'

I suppose that's fair enough. 'Once I explained that it would be better having its own food I think the laddie was happy. In fact I think once he realised that he wouldn't have to give any more of his chocolate away he was quite happy!'

ALTHOUGH IT WAS now nearly nine o'clock, this gentle operation was almost therapeutic at the end of the day and I'd hardly noticed the time.

'I'll finish off here, Willie. You'd better go home and get something to eat.'

'Oh it's all right. I'm in no hurry.'

'Well, we'll have a wee dram before you go, then. Right, that's you fixed up, wee dog. Can you put it in the recovery room while I clean up, Willie?'

The recovery room is our rather grand name for a small heated room (originally the maid's lavatory) kept warm with an infra-red lamp. Animals recovering from an operation get put in there while they come round. It keeps the body temperature up while they get over the anaesthetic.

'Make sure you close the door properly.' I'm not afraid to remind everyone about that. Just after we'd made the room years ago I put a cat in there to recover from being spayed. I went into the kitchen to do the books and completely forgot about it. When the owner came to collect it later on, I went into the room and it had gone. I searched the storeroom next door, behind all the boxes and bottles. Nothing. I looked into the kitchen and the living room. Still no sign of the animal. I had to tell the owner that it hadn't quite recovered from the anaesthetic and ask him to call back again later. Meanwhile we continued the search, eventually finding the cat under one of the girls' beds. The last time the cat had seen me I'd stuck a needle in her, so she was understandably unwilling to make my acquaintance again. In the end Jane had to coax her out.

I POURED TWO glasses of whisky and a vodka for Jane. The three of us sat in the kitchen and chatted for a while. Jane said that there'd been a call from someone in Aviemore who wanted to bring their budgerigar into the surgery tomorrow. She and Willie smiled at the thought of this, knowing what had happened once when I had dealings with a bird of that species, It must have been a while ago now. This man, a big strapping chap, came in with a green-and-white budgie in a cage. He was slightly embarrassed and explained that it was his wife's pet which she'd had for a long time. It needed its claws cut and his wife, he said, couldn't bear to see it in pain, and had stayed outside just in case it suffered when I did it. I thought that was a bit odd – after all, cutting the claws is hardly a major operation – but then some people get very upset if they think their animal's suffering in the slightest. From the grudging tone of his voice it wasn't hard to guess that there was no love lost between him and the bird.

I looked at the bird inside the cage. It looked pretty healthy and I told him I thought it would live for ages. I asked the chap to reach in and hold it while I put the light on. As I turned I heard the cage open. 'Come on then, you poor little beggar.'

I told him to hold on to it – I didn't fancy having to chase it around the surgery all evening. But there didn't seem any chance of that; he couldn't get hold of it at all. Even though it was only a small cage the bird was fluttering around trying to avoid capture. I told him to move out of the way and let me get it. I reached in and managed to get my hand around the bird. With the clippers in one hand and the budgie in the other, I moved across to the light, for a clearer view of what I was doing.

As I bent over to look, I thought there was something not quite right, but couldn't work out what it was. Then I realised. There was no movement from the tiny body. Not a flicker. It had died, there and then in the surgery.

The man seemed unaware that there was anything wrong. He was probably thinking about getting the job over so that he could get back to the pub.

I straightened up, knowing that there was no easy way of breaking the news.

'You're not going to believe this. I'm afraid it's dead.' The simple statement had more effect than I could have imagined. He looked first at me, then the green-and-yellow ball of feathers in my hand, then back at me. He looked as though he'd seen all the ghosts from the battle of Culloden Moor in the surgery. He still didn't say a word, but went white. From his look I thought he was going to be my next patient.

'I'm afraid the shock of having your hand then mine coming into the cage must have been too much for him,' I explained. 'I think he just died of fright.' But he wasn't really listening; he was far away.

Suddenly he pulled himself together and blurted out, 'For God's sake, can't you give it an injection or something and bring it back to life? My wife'll kill me!' He meant it as well. 'You've got to do something. You don't realise how serious this is.' I was tempted to say that it was pretty serious for the budgie too but luckily managed to restrain myself. 'I can't go out and tell her that it's dead. She'll never believe I didn't do it on purpose!'

I think it was one of the rare occasions when I've witnessed real panic at close quarters. Don't let anyone ever say that women are less powerful than men – looking at this husband and the fear in his eyes I think I know who I'd have put money on in a power struggle in their relationship.

'Can't you give it an injection or something?' He really couldn't believe that there was nothing I could do. In those few moments he'd become a desperate man. 'You'll have to keep it in overnight.' I was about to explain that even twenty-four hours of concentrated vetting were unlikely to strengthen my powers of healing to the extent of bringing things back from the dead, when he continued. 'I'll have to go out tomorrow and buy another one.'

Now in times of stress people behave strangely and I thought it prudent to point out that she'd probably notice the difference. 'I'll say that you've given it some drugs which change the feathers or something.'

Well the man left and came back the next day to pick up the cage. They've never been back here with the new one. I can only assume that the wifee didn't notice any difference. I just hope that she thought I'd done a good job, and that the budgie lived to a ripe old age. She probably ended up by thinking that her pet held the world age record for budgies.

I hope nothing similar happens with tomorrow's patient. Perhaps I'll let Willie take care of it.

IT WAS ABOUT half past nine when Willie left, having had his dram. For both of us, fourteen-hour days are pretty normal, and when you enjoy what you're doing it's no real hardship. As I sit here in the kitchen writing, Jane is in the lounge knitting as she does most nights. Even though it's August there's a peat fire burning. I like to have that going most of the year. We don't have any central heating in the house and because it's made from local granite it takes a lot of heating up, so the open fire in the front room and the Esse stove in the kitchen are kept going all year round. I have my own peat moss on one of the nearby hills, and I suppose cutting the peat each year is one of my few hobbies. It's the only kind of leisure pursuit I can cope with because it has a practical use – I get the enjoyment of digging hard for a few hours and the satisfaction of knowing that I'm providing fuel at the same time. As they say around here, with peat you get two heats, one digging it and the other burning it.

THURSDAY 18 AUGUST

THIS MORNING I called on a patient who's been giving me a few problems lately, an Arctic fox. It's one of the animals at the Highland Wildlife Park, just outside Aviemore. It has some sort of bad throat infection which we've not been able to identify so far. I gave it another injection of penicillin, and we put it back into the isolation cage in the park's sick bay.

There's an air of change at the park at the moment. The head keeper is leaving to sail in the Mediterranean, and the man who started it all up, Eddie Orbell, is retiring. The project was born in 1971, when a group of businessmen came up with the idea of providing somewhere for indigenous Scottish animals to be put on show. Like many of these projects it grew to include any animals which had become extinct in Scotland, but were known to have lived here up to 10 000 years ago.

Initially most of the collection came from Scotland, some from England, and the European bison were imported from Poland, Sweden and Denmark. They didn't seem to mind the change of nationality and bred quite well. I think a couple of the originals are still there, and some of their progeny have gone off to stock other collections.

I was never actually asked to become their vet, but as usually happens in the area I got to hear that something was afoot. Thinking that I was in danger of being asked to treat some strange beast, I ordered copies of textbooks dealing with exotic animals in captivity. They proved to be a worthwhile investment. It wasn't long before I had a call to ask if I would look at a golden eagle with a bad leg. In the end I just sort of drifted into being their vet. Now they've everything from wolves, wild boars and wildcats to pine martens, capercaillie and brown bears. It's provided me with many interesting and unusual cases to treat over the years.

Eddie was clearing his desk when I called in on him and inevitably we got talking about some of the animals we've treated together, often in unusual circumstances. One wild exhibit arrived and turned out not to be quite so wild as we'd been led to believe.

For some years there had been reports of cattle, sheep and even foals being attacked in the district by a large cat-like creature. Then one day I got a call from Eddie at the Wildlife Park to say that they thought the culprit had been found. Someone had phoned the press to say that they'd found a puma caught in a trap. Eddie was taking it into the park, and wanted me to have a look at the leg which they thought had been damaged when the trap shut on it.

When I arrived, the puma was pacing up and down in a small cage. There were quite a few park staff watching, but no one ventured anywhere near, in case it became vicious and lashed out at them. It was obviously lame and we wanted to check that there was nothing wrong in the leg or foot that would require treatment. There was no way that I was going into the cage until the animal was sedated, so I loaded my gun with the special dart containing anaesthetic, and fired it straight into the animal's backside.

While we watched the puma getting sleepier, there was a general discussion about the best type of permanent cage to keep it in, because obviously we didn't want to endanger any members of the staff or viewing public in any way. When it was out cold we went into the cage and weighed it, I think it weighed about 81 pounds which was pretty heavy for a puma. It was in pretty good condition overall, even though we could see from its teeth that it wasn't in the first flush of youth. I took samples of its faeces and sent them off to see if we could discover what it had been feeding on. All the time I was in there I kept saying to Eddie, 'Be sure and tell me if it thinks about coming round.' I didn't want to be forced to make friends with a puma suffering from a sore head.

The leg was not really damaged and there was nothing much we could do, so we left the puma in the cage, making sure to double lock it, while it came round. Several newspapers ran stories about this wild animal which had been captured, and everyone believed that the mystery of the animal deaths over the previous few years had been solved. They were also full of speculation as to where it might have come from. Various theories were proffered including one suggestion that it had been a stowaway which had jumped ship in the North Sea and swum ashore.

After a few days, though, the keeper looking after it noticed that it didn't seem very vicious. He'd been into the cage to feed it and said that it actually seemed to like the company. At the same time the results of the sample analysis came back, revealing that it had been fed on cat food and other domestic foodstuffs. We all started to smell a rat, and realised that we'd been done. It became clear that the puma had been a pet, which presumably had grown too big. Its owners had disposed of it, just as other people dump dogs, in the middle of nowhere. More disturbing than that, the owners must have put it into the trap and then rung the press with the wild puma story.

As time wore on the keeper really got friendly with it, and it never attempted to attack him. Occasionally it would take his leg in its mouth, but only in play – it never bit him. It would also jump up on to his shoulders in an act of affection, although this proved to be a bit on the dangerous side because it had the habit of digging its claws in to get a grip, and they would go straight through the jacket into his flesh. I went over to see it one day and took my granddaughter with me. We went into the cage together and it rubbed itself up against her like a big pussy cat. It settled in very happily at the Wildlife Park and became quite an attraction. In fact it only died a couple of years ago

It's often occurred to me that the people who visit the park are the creatures in captivity as they drive around with their car doors shut, while the animals roam free over acres of land. Some of the animals, such as the bison, can get a bit frisky if they get too close to humans, so there are strict rules designed to keep visitors safe. They're told not to get out of the car, or lower the windows. But despite all the warnings there have been times when stubborn or stupid visitors have left the safety of their vehicle and caused problems.

There was a roe deer in the park which had been hand reared and consequently had no fear of people. It was very pretty to look at and deceptively docile in appearance. It was introduced into the drive-through section of the park. One visitor insisted on getting out of his car to get his camera from the boot to take a picture of it. A ranger saw him and told him to return to the car at once. The man refused, insisting that he got his camera. The ranger had another go, seeing the roe deer approaching at great speed, head lowered and sharp horns poised for action. The next thing the gentleman knew he was inside the boot of the car. The deer had given him a good whack up the backside and tipped him over the edge.

Another day Eddie was driving into the enclosed area when he saw a lady already inside, happily strolling across the paddock, camera in hand, towards the fence, probably to take a picture of some of the strange dark-brown motheaten-looking Mouflon sheep. It was a bright, hot summer's day and she was wearing a short-sleeved top. Before Eddie could get close enough to shout, she leaned her forearms on the fence ... and gave the most enormous shout of surprise, followed almost immediately by a cry of pain. The fence is electrified and she'd got a few volts through her when she touched it.

But to add insult to injury the roe deer had strolled up behind her and, possibly excited by the sudden movement and sound, butted her. Her husband, who had remained in the car, saw all

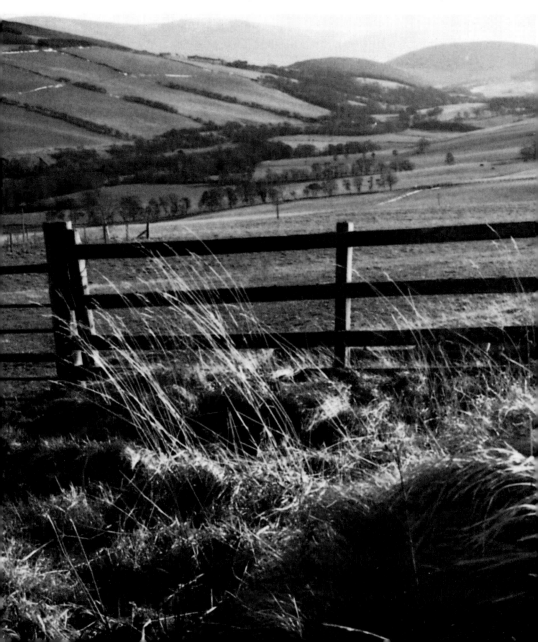

this and made a gallant but ill-advised rescue attempt. The roe deer saw the man running towards him, thought this was great sport and promptly attacked him too.

Instead of leaving his aggressor alone the man thought he'd play Tarzan and try to catch the deer, who by this time must have thought he was being given a new toy to play with. The ranger shouted at him to get back in the car, but he insisted on completing his mission. It all happened in a few moments, before anyone else could stop him. To give him his due he managed to

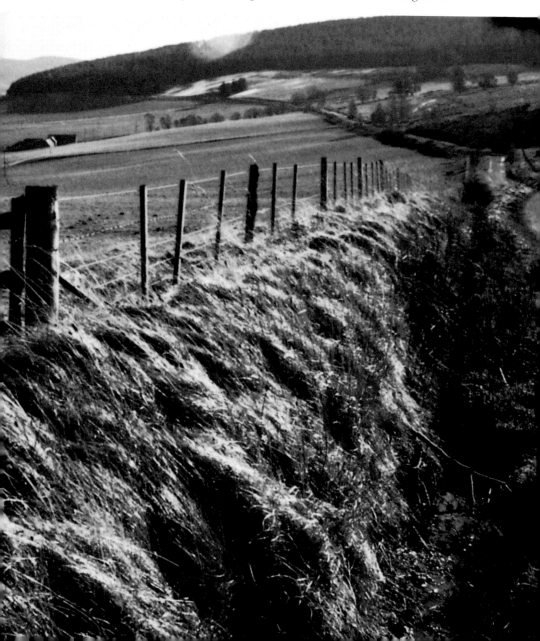

get hold of the horns and let his wife back into the car before getting in himself. However I'm sure if he'd just got back in the car, the deer would have lost interest and wandered off. The hero escaped with only a few superficial cuts and bruises and the couple later apologised profusely for their stupidity.

That roe deer attacked about fourteen people in all, none of them seriously. All of the victims admitted that it was their own fault for getting out of their cars to go and stroke this nice little Bambi lookalike, who actually had a playful temperament, but the wherewithal to do some damage.

I have to say that it was seldom the animals who caused the problems – almost always the humans. I was there another day when there was a shout from one of the badger's nocturnal enclosures and a man came running out with his trousers in disarray. 'Good God, it's full of bloody skunks,' he cried. 'I thought it was the gents' toilets.'

In the park's office there's a reminder of another close scrape, in the shape of a small Polaroid photograph. They were running a photographic competition one year and a man approached one of the wardens, holding this picture in his hand, to ask if it could be entered in the competition. When the warden looked, it was of the man's son, standing underneath the full grown bull bison. The boy had a broad grin on his face, and was holding a piece of white sliced bread up to its mouth to feed it. We often look at it and think ignorance is bliss.

I was injecting an otter one day when a lady started to complain to Eddie about an outrageous spectacle she'd just witnessed. One of the wardens, Donald Mitchell, was a true Scotsman, and quite frequently wore his kilt on duty. There was a goat in one of the pens which would regularly put its head through the fence and then get its horns stuck. Donald had gone over and pulled and heaved with all his might until the goat came loose and they both flew backwards, landing in a heap, exposing all of Donald's manhood to the onlookers. The lady said she had brought a group of children on a visit, and though, she assured Eddie, she wasn't a prude, she thought that in the interests of decency his staff ought to wear something underneath their traditional attire, especially with so many young children about. How we stopped laughing I have no idea. As she was berating him, we could see her group of children behind her taking great pleasure in watching a pair of deer mating!

AMONG THE MOST popular exhibits at the park are their brown bears. And it was one of the bears that was the cause of perhaps the most exciting adventure I've been involved in.

Back in 1976 I had a call from Eddie to say that they'd sold a bear cub to a chap called Andy Robin. I recognised the name: he was a wrestler who had been all over the world performing. Apparently he'd been in Canada and had been matched against a wrestling bear called 'Terrible Ted', which had been muzzled and chained. He decided that one day he would bring up a bear in such a way that it would live with him and eventually wrestle in the ring without being restrained in any way. I often wonder what makes people decide to make a living from something like that! Andy had heard that one of the bears at the Highland Wildlife Park was pregnant, and had been in negotiation with Eddie about buying one of the cubs. Eddie must have grilled him at length, and been satisfied that Andy would give it a good home, or else I'm sure he wouldn't have agreed to a deal.

In the end Andy bought a ten-month-old, 13-stone 'baby' for £50, and Hercules' career was launched. I was called upon to sedate it so that it could be moved into a crate and taken away. We managed to get the drug into the cub, and the cub into the crate. Hercules was taken away and that was the last I expected to see of him, in the fur at least.

Over the next couple of years I read the odd article about Hercules, and he and Andy appeared in wrestling matches on television. At one point he starred in a TV commercial advertising toilet rolls. It was amazing to see how quickly that cuddly cub had grown into a 54-stone, 9-foot-high grizzly bear! I never dreamt that our paths would cross again in a dramatic way several years later.

One evening in August 1980, I received one of those phone calls which start innocently enough, but develop into something extraordinary. Having established that I was Mr George Rafferty, veterinary surgeon, the voice on the end of the line told me to 'wait one please'. Which in itself was rather a strange form of words, but gave a clue to the official nature of the call. Then the line went dead for a second and a different voice started to speak. 'Hello, Mr Rafferty, this is the Chief Constable.'

That's it, I thought. I've been found out at last. What terrible misdemeanour had I committed which warranted a personal call from the top man? Could it be that I'd been seen stopping on the double yellow line outside the paper shop to pick up my *Financial Times*? Or had my heinous crime of forty years ago been discovered, when as a student I pinched a flower from the graveyard, on my way to a date? I wasn't left in suspense for very long. 'Can you get your things together and fly over to the island of Benbecula in the Hebrides?' he asked. This was a strange request, but more was to come. 'Hercules has escaped and is loose on the island.'

I didn't immediately connect the name with nearly 1000 pounds of grizzly bear. Then as the Chief Constable continued it clicked, and a picture built up in my mind of this huge beast running wild amongst masses of people. 'Could you get over to the island and help catch him?' was the Chief Constable's simple request.

I've never been one to get on the wrong side of any policeman, especially not one of such high rank, so I started packing straight away. The main priority was the dart gun and enough drugs to have several attempts at darting Hercules if necessary. The Chief Constable had also asked Eddie Orbell to go along.

I think we felt like two schoolboys setting off on an adventure. It was a terribly stormy day and all we'd been told was to report as soon as possible to Inverness airport, where our transport would be waiting. In the rush to get ready, the full implications of this hadn't dawned on me. It was only when we listened to the radio on the way to the airport and heard the news, that the reality started to sink in.

All the boats in the Hebrides had put into port to shelter from a fierce storm, which was presumably why the Chief Constable had said that we had no choice in our means of transport. Now I'd never flown before, and it wasn't an aspect of modern life I'd had any desire to experience. I certainly wouldn't have chosen a day when the weather was so bad that hardy seamen had given up and sought shelter. We got talking about this and I ventured an opinion, which I freely admitted to Eddie was nothing more than a gut feeling: if the weather was so bad that sea transport wasn't able to cope, I suggested, wouldn't the air be even more drastically affected, especially at the low altitudes we would presumably be flying at for our brief hop across Scotland. On this day we had no choice, however. We were needed in a hurry, we had to fly, and, well, we were in it too deep now to back out.

By the time we got to the airport, the outing which had started as a pleasant jaunt for the boys was suddenly looking a bit more serious. Then, as we turned into the car park, we saw what, to me, seemed like a huge jet airliner sitting on the tarmac. Right away, I felt a bit more secure.

We were met by a policeman, who said that all the arrangements had been completed and were to go straight to the plane. Obviously others also jumped when the Chief Constable was involved. He introduced us to a lady in uniform who, he said, would look after us. I thought that things were looking up again. At least we'd have some pleasant female company to take our minds off the horrors of flying in bumpy weather. She told us to make our way to the plane, she just had to pick up some papers, and then we could leave. We walked out on to the tarmac, where the wind was really quite strong, and moved towards the big jet. Then I heard the woman's voice, 'No not that way, over here.'

Strange, I thought, there must be another one around the corner. Then one of those blinding moments of realisation occurred. She was walking towards the tiniest plane I have ever seen. Worse than that, and you'll have to forgive my old-fashioned Highland ways, *she* got into the driving seat, and started to flick all the switches. This was, I thought to myself, the time to suddenly remember a pressing engagement back in my nice, safe, warm surgery in Grantown.

It was too late for chickening out, though. There was just room for the three of us and our equipment inside the plane. Looking at Eddie I could see that he was in a similar state of shock at the events unfolding around us. By this time the engine was revving up and we were taxiing down the runway.

The flight was a bit bumpy, but surprisingly neither of us was ill. I think we were in a state of disbelief about the whole thing. Only a few hours earlier I'd been looking forward to a day of routine calls, now here we were flying out to the Hebrides in the middle of a storm.

We landed safely, and I have to say that she was a marvellous pilot. We were greeted on the island by the head of the local police who took us to a hotel where I met my counterpart on Benbecula, the vet Pat Ford. Eventually a message arrived saying that something had been seen not far from where Hercules had escaped, so we rushed off to the point where the bear had disappeared, but after looking for a while found nothing. Andy Robin was up in a helicopter looking all over the islands, but was having no luck either. He touched down briefly to see us, but was soon off again.

There wasn't much we could do so we went back to the hotel to wait; then, when darkness fell, we moved camp to Pat Ford's house where we spent the night. He was able to fill us in on how Hercules came to be loose on the island. Apparently Andy and his wife Maggie had gone to Benbecula for a holiday, taking Hercules with them in the back of the customised coach the three of them used to travel about in. They'd been enjoying taking Hercules swimming in the sea every day and generally having a great time. But a few days into the holiday Hercules had decided to swim off, and Andy had watched helplessly as he disappeared out to sea, only to turn back in to land far in the distance, and lumber off with Andy in pursuit. He was last seen swimming across to one of the smaller islands, called Wiay.

The next day the plan was to invade Wiay with army personnel from the rocket range in Benbecula. Eddie and I started to feel like adventurers again. We were taken over to the island in an army rubber assault boat, and we spent the day searching the mile or so of land with the soldiers. We didn't see any sign of Hercules, who must have been biding his time somewhere. It was a bit frustrating to have had all the excitement of the journey there and then the landing on the island, without actually achieving anything, but there wasn't much any of us could do. At the end of the second day we held a meeting and it was decided that there wasn't much point in us staying, so regretfully we returned to Inverness and home.

Andy and Maggie kept up the search for days on end with amazing dedication and stamina. They found the odd paw print here and there, but there was no sign of the bear himself. I must admit I wondered if he had drowned attempting to swim for one of the other islands, and I thought we'd heard the last of Hercules.

I went back to the routine work of the practice, which for a while was a bit of an anti-climax. Every now and again the radio and the television would carry a brief story mentioning that the bear was still loose somewhere in the islands, but it was largely forgotten.

Then about three weeks after the first phone call, the police phoned again with an even more urgent request for help. Hercules had been spotted on North Uist. They asked if we could go out either to dart and anaesthetise him, or, if that wasn't possible, to shoot him. The police were worried that now he was on an inhabited island again, and presumably pretty hungry, he might attack somebody. I think that would have been highly unlikely, but I suppose they had to take that line just to be on the safe side.

With all the press interest in the affair, I didn't relish the thought that I might have to be the one to kill Hercules, who by now had become a national hero. By coincidence a chap called Alan Mann who ran a helicopter company was in the north of Scotland on a week's deerstalking. When he heard about the bear on the loose he'd put his helicopter at the disposal of the police, so he ended up flying over to fetch us.

Flying in a helicopter was another first for me and quite a different experience. Alan, with his co-pilot John Ackroyd-Hunt, picked us up just outside Grantown, and flew us to the island. It was a great thrill to fly along the course of the River Spey and have a bird's-eye view of all the farms in the practice which I knew so well. As we flew over the hills I could see the shielings where the cows used to be sent in the summer. Then over the Cuillins in Skye. I couldn't get over how sharp they were; my admiration increased for anyone who climbs up there.

When we arrived at Benbecula, the airport was seething with planes. It seemed that press from all over the world were there. The fact that Hercules had turned up after three weeks on the loose had made him a really good story when everyone, including me, had presumed that he had swum out to sea and had drowned. We went into the control tower and met Andy Robin. He was understandably in quite a state by now, and had been interviewed by every conceivable press person. It was probably a good thing, therefore, that there wasn't room in the helicopter to take Andy as well as us.

On our way out to the helicopter, Andy came up to me, fixed me with a hard stare and said fiercely, 'Just you make sure you don't kill the bugger.' Andy had been British Commonwealth Wrestling Champion, and even after the exertions of the previous three weeks he was a big chap. I was quite sure that if we killed the bear Andy Robin would make sure that a similar fate would befall us. So as we boarded the helicopter again I said to the pilot, 'If we do kill this bear we're going to fly right back to the mainland and take no chances. We're not going to risk coming back to Benbecula to face Andy.'

The operation had been carefully planned and we flew up and down North Uist in a set pattern, backwards and forwards, with four pairs of eyes straining for any sign of our prey. There had been farms in this particularly desolate part of North Uist in the old days, but they had long been empty, and only the skeletons of the buildings remained. Whenever we came to one of these derelict places we would land, and I had the task of getting out of the helicopter and walking into each building in turn to search them. I noticed that the other faces in the cabin managed to hide any traces of disappointment that I was the one to undertake this enviable part of our task.

It was quite eerie, and I was a bit apprehensive every time I had to creep around a corner in case the bear was on the other side in a bad mood, and decided to clobber me. After all, he had been on the run for quite a while, and might have got used to his own company. Worse than that, he might have got a bit confused as to the distinction between friend and food. It was just like a scene from a horror film, except that the heroes in the cinema have the assistance of music which plays louder as a warning when something is going to happen. Out there on my own, the only sound was the distant whirring of the helicopter blades and the creak of old timbers. I don't mind admitting to a tingling sensation down my spine at each unexplained noise.

Fortunately Hercules wasn't in any of the buildings and we took off again. Then suddenly the pilot saw him out in the open. He heard the helicopter and set off in the opposite direction. We watched as he ran into a wee loch and started swimming, but there was nowhere he could go so we landed in order to load the darts. While we were doing that we radioed back with the good news of our sightings. There was a joyful scream from Andy at the other end. We told the press to keep back in all their planes so that they didn't frighten him. I was using a powerful anaesthetic which can be lethal to humans, so it was quite tricky working in the confined space of the helicopter. If I'd knocked the pilot out we'd have been stranded. The other problem was that we'd been told that Hercules weighed 54 stone when he got away, but I was worried that he'd have lost weight during his period roaming free. I didn't want to overdose him and kill him.

I calculated a dose based on all these factors, filled some brand new darts, and completed my preparations by loading them into the gun. Which was when I discovered that I might have a major, very public problem on my hands. The new darts were too big for the gun. So we had to split the dose, half in a smaller dart and the rest in a syringe which someone, no prizes for guessing who, would have to inject into the bear, which made it even more tricky.

At last we were ready to take off again to find Hercules. We flew for a minute or so before we saw him. The pilot, Captain John Ackroyd-Hunt, was superb. He'd spent nine years in Africa tracking and capturing game, and it showed in the way he handled the helicopter.

Eddie took the first shot, but the downdraught from the rotors blew it off course. So the Captain said that next time Eddie was ready, he was to shout 'Now!' and he would momentarily reduce the downdraught while the gun was fired. Hercules had an idea that something was about to happen and took off at a fair lick up a hillside trying to escape from the helicopter. We caught up with him; Eddie lined up the sights of the rifle, and shouted 'Now!'; the pilot trimmed the blades; I held my breath. Eddie fired. And the dart found its home in the bear's backside.

He didn't fall straight away but started to run. We followed him at a distance so as not to frighten him even more. Then he started to stagger and eventually got really weary, and ran down into a ravine, at the bottom of which was a little stream or burn.

We landed and Eddie and I ran up the hill to see what had happened. We peered down into the ravine, where we saw Hercules lying across the burn. I was afraid that he'd dam the water and drown himself, so I got a rope from the helicopter and lassoed him around the neck, thinking that if worse came to worst we could drag him out with the helicopter. There was no other way that we'd have been able to attempt it.

But Hercules must have felt the rope, because suddenly he was up and off again. I tried desperately to hold on to him, but there was no way I could do anything. It was like trying to hold back a train. It must have been quite a sight, me being dragged across the scrubland and up the hillside by this huge bear. They didn't teach us anything about this at veterinary college.

My weight on the rope had some effect, though. Hercules became increasingly tired and eventually he fell again. I'd been carrying the other dose of anaesthetic in a syringe tucked behind my ear, and I crept up behind him and stuck it into his backside. After about five minutes he completely collapsed.

With a final burst of energy on our part we rolled him into a net which we tied together and slung beneath the helicopter on a special hook. Hercules had been recaptured after twenty-four days on the loose. We took off and flew back at 100 miles an hour with the bear swinging beneath us, hanging by this one hook.

Eddie had to be left behind because we were carrying so much extra weight, and he told me later that as we took off he noticed that the hook wasn't closed properly. He said that he tried to attract our attention and stop us, but we all thought he was just waving his fond farewells. It turned out that the hook hadn't shut automatically as it should have done, and it was only the wind resistance that kept the net in place. I never dared tell Andy that!

When we landed they put the bear in a pick-up truck, and took him back to the bus which was absolutely full of reporters making a heck of a noise. Andy was in tears at seeing his old friend again; his wife Maggie was overcome. About eight people carried Hercules into his quarters in the bus and I was a bit afraid to revive him because of all the excitement. The last time I'd darted and revived the bear he'd been a sixth of the size he was now, and

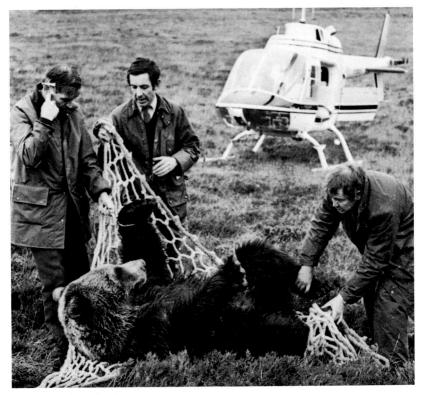

Hercules captured at last.

I couldn't tell how grizzly this grizzly would be. Some animals become aggressive after they've been given this particular drug and been revived, and I didn't want anything to go wrong. So instead of giving the antidote intravenously, I gave it to him in his backside so that it took effect slowly. He came around gently and placidly and he seemed right as rain.

As soon as I was satisfied that he wasn't hurt, we had to leave. The weather was really closing in by then, and Alan Mann and John Ackroyd-Hunt wanted to be back on the mainland before it was pitch black.

My reward for those exploits was a letter of commendation from the Chief Constable and a case of champagne from Maggie, Andy and Hercules. I don't drink champagne much so I swopped it for a case of whisky. I think I got the best of the bargain.

Somewhere on the spot where it all happened will be a camera complete with a roll of undeveloped film. I had it in my pocket and it must have fallen out at some stage of the operation. It will still be lying there with some unique snaps. Alan Mann took quite a few pictures, but I was the only one near to Hercules before he was knocked out – the others kept their distance until he was well and truly sedated.

ABOUT A YEAR after the Hercules affair, and probably as a result of the publicity surrounding our exploits, Eddie and I were asked if we would take part in another adventure. An American film company was over in Glencoe making a film called *In Quest of Fire* in which three lions were to appear. Their insurance company had insisted that a veterinary surgeon and an animal handler should be present during the relevant sequences, with a dart gun to tranquillise the lions if necessary, and a rifle should more drastic action be required.

I was quite delighted to go, and pleased that Eddie Orbell would be with me. When the film company asked what our fee would be, I more or less plucked a figure out of the air of £100 a day plus expenses, which I thought would be a pretty good day's wage to split between us. This was accepted, and we went down to Fort William complete with rifle and dart gun.

We had been told to report to a particular hotel where the film unit had based themselves, and, sure enough, there were two rooms booked for us. I must admit that it felt like a holiday to us and we sauntered into the bar ready for a pleasant evening. In my days in Glasgow I was used to having to make my way to the bar through some pretty hefty chaps, but here we were confronted with some of the biggest men I have ever seen. They turned out to be wrestlers from America who had been flown over to play the part of cavemen in the film. Towards the end of the evening one of them took a chap who must have weighed all of 12 stone and with one hand lifted him up on top of the bar.

We didn't meet anyone from the production unit that evening, but letters were pushed under our bedroom doors during the night instructing us to be at the location by eight o'clock the following morning.

When we went down for breakfast, I was surprised that only one other table was occupied. Thinking about the antics of the previous night, we assumed they'd all had too much to drink, and couldn't face food. So Eddie and I set off in the car for Glencoe and found the location.

It was an amazing set-up, like an army on manoeuvres, with tracked vehicles on site to convey the numerous people involved in the action across a very boggy moor. When we jumped down from the transport we were confronted by a hive of activity, with masses of people milling around yet more wagons, a couple of marquees and technical equipment such as generators and cranes.

I could see why they'd chosen the spot. It was really beautiful, on the edge of a loch, with a lone tree standing by the edge of the water. We were introduced to Dickie and Jimmy Chipperfield, the circus people, who'd supplied the animals. Over the next few days we came to know them quite well as delightful people, full of great stories of their exploits in the circus world. The Chipperfields' three lions were going to be turned into sabre-toothed tigers, which was to be achieved by gluing great long plastic extensions on to their canine teeth. Getting the teeth on took some doing, I can tell you, but the Chipperfields were fearless people and took it in their stride. I would definitely not have volunteered for the job.

I then discovered why no one had been down to breakfast that morning. The film company had told me that they would pay for our room in the hotel, and would give us a daily allowance of £3.50 for breakfast, £11 for dinner, plus £2 for location expenses. But at nine o'clock at the location there was a bus fitted up as a restaurant complete with tables, where they served coffee and rolls with ham and eggs, as much as you could eat. At lunch there was a four-course meal provided free – real lavish food such as roast beef with all the trimmings – all cooked up in the back of a specially converted lorry. And finally at teatime there were as many cakes as you could stuff into yourself. So everyone but us had waited for food until they were on location, when they knew it would be possible to eat as much as they wanted without having to touch the daily cash handout.

As Eddie and I were digging into the mound of food, a flustered and worried-looking assistant director came up to us and described how the scene would run. The sabre-toothed tigers would chase some cavemen towards the loch. The men would climb up the tree and the lions would jump at them in their place of refuge, and try to claw them down. The Chipperfields had devised an ingenious method of achieving this which was to lay a trail of meat up to the tree, which the lions were to run along. Then they would jump up and claw at lumps of meat hung just beneath where the cavemen would be clinging. The meat, of course, would be carefully concealed, so it would look as though they were trying to grab at the men's legs.

This all sounded plausible, and Jimmy Chipperfield assured us that there would be no problem with the animals attacking the cavemen. The big, hairy wrestlers I'd seen flexing their muscles last night thought different. They refused to play the game. So it was left to the Chipperfields' lion attendants to strip off to bare essentials and run the course clad only in the briefest of caveman costumes. They were more worried by the possible effects of the October temperatures than the fear of being savaged by the ferocious animals. With each successive take of the action the stand-ins who'd found exposure of more than one kind thrust upon them seemed to become more exuberant. It might have had something to do with the way they were revived after each take with a drop of brandy.

Precautions had been taken to ensure everyone else's safety. There were cages for anybody who had to be on the set during the filming, so all we were really concerned with was what would happen if the lions decided to make a bid for freedom. To dissuade them from this course of action, a huge fence had been erected around three sides of the area; the fourth being bounded by the loch. The assistant director seemed really pleased with this arrangement, and even more pleased with the vantage point which had been provided for us. Eddie and I were to be about halfway along the area on a platform which they'd built specially.

We listened to the explanation and looked at each other. I said that I thought the two of us ought to walk around the set and examine it more closely. We moved away, trying to look as though we were assessing our lines of sight, testing the strength of the fence, and generally attempting to give the impression that we were earning our vast fee. In fact as soon as we were out of earshot of the film people we had a conversation which went something like this:

EDDIE   'The lions could easily get round the fence where it goes into the water.'

ME   'We haven't got a hope of hitting anything from that platform if they get away.'
(More gesticulation and apparent intense measuring.)

EDDIE   'Seems a bit of a shame to stop their filming, though, with all this money being spent.'
(Reassuring wave to the assistant director, who is now running around like a headless chicken.)

ME   'They wouldn't get any further than the bog whatever happened, would they?'

Without many more words passing between us we came to a decision. We casually sauntered back towards the platform, attempting to create the illusion that we had simply confirmed our plan of action, and that we were totally in control of the situation. We mumbled 'Fine' and 'Aye, Laddie' a few times to the assistant director who looked as though any sign of doubt on our part would have been the final straw, then we sloped off to see the Chipperfields.

We mentioned quietly to the Chipperfields our doubts about the effectiveness of the precautions against escape. They assured us that lions didn't like water, so they wouldn't swim for it. I still wasn't completely convinced – the water was very shallow, and I was sure that any lion could have walked into it and around the side of the fence. But Dickie Chipperfield was completely relaxed about the whole thing, and all he said was, 'If they do try to escape, be sure to dart the big lion. It's very valuable because it does a trick where the trainer puts his head in its mouth. The others are just ordinary ones – you can do what you like to them if they get away.'

I didn't think it was prudent to tell him that the lions would have been pretty safe whichever weapon we used! Eddie and I had a sort of conference and concluded that we hadn't any hope of hitting them if they escaped. All we'd be able to do would be to phone Alan Mann and get his helicopter up! However we decided that the Chipperfields were the experts and we'd take their advice.

As it turned out our fears were groundless. The filming went on for about three days during which time the lions behaved impeccably. Which was lucky for us – it would have been a bit embarrassing to have had to stand by and watch them run off into the distance.

What I couldn't get over was the way money was spent as though it was going out of fashion. If they needed more mini-buses or tracked vehicles they just phoned down to Edinburgh and had them sent up. I suppose it seemed even more amazing to me because I'd been so used to working with farmers who watched every penny they spent.

This extravagance was brought home very clearly to me on the second day when at about eight o'clock in the morning Dickie Chipperfield came up to me in a real panic and asked if I could get him two wild rabbits. Apparently the script called for the cavemen to chase two rabbits, catch them and skin them. They then had to eat them raw, because they weren't supposed to have any method of cooking. The Chipperfields had brought two rabbits from their safari park with them, and when it came to the point at which the rabbits were required, they'd let them out of their cage and set the cavemen running after them. But unfortunately, instead of dashing off with the actors in hot pursuit, the rabbits had turned, run towards their supposed aggressors, and stood there waiting to be stroked. No one had taken into account that they were tame, and used to being handled. In the end they had had to abandon the scene, but they wanted to try it again at three o'clock that afternoon. In order to capture two wild rabbits by then, I needed to unearth one tame ferret, which could be put down a burrow to bolt the rabbits out into a waiting net.

Not knowing anyone in the district I set off down the road to a house which I thought looked like a keeper's house, and hammered on the door for ages. Eventually this big chap, looking extremely bleary eyed, came to the door and I asked him if he was a keeper. He wasn't, of course, but he pointed me in the direction of the nearest one. It was only as I walked away that I realised I'd woken up Hamish MacInnes, the famous mountaineer.

I found the keeper's house, and asked for his help. He said

no one in the area had a ferret, so I thought the only thing to do was to phone a friend in Grantown who kept a ferret and ask him to go out and catch the rabbits for me.

Well at 2.55 I thought we'd blown it, when all of a sudden the chap's sister turned up with one rabbit. She said that the ferret had got two but had eaten one of them. Anyway, I produced the one rabbit and they paid her £70. We hung around for a while but in the end were told that they were running late because of the weather, and they wouldn't get to it that day. I had to go back to Grantown, so someone from the film company took the rabbit back to the hotel in one of my wire cat baskets. I heard later that when they went to fetch the star the following morning it was dead. They'd left it in a room in the hotel which had been too hot. So they wasted their money *and* had to get another one.

When the filming of the lions was finished our services were dispensed with, and we were sent to the accountant to be paid. He sat in one of the hotel rooms behind a table piled high with these special cash boxes full of money. He confirmed that the agreement was for £100 a day and passed us each an envelope. We thanked him very much, and left. It was only when we got home and counted the money that we discovered we'd been paid a £100 a day *each*. They must have misunderstood my original statement, but if they thought we were worth that much, who was I to disagree.

AS IT TURNED out those weren't our last dealings with them. After the filming was finished in Glencoe they moved up to Strathspey and were joined by several elephants which were to play the part of hairy mammoths. To disguise them, the film company had provided big cloaks with hair on them, and tusks which they'd stuck on as extensions to the real thing. I saw them after they'd been made up, before they went off into the hills, and they looked very realistic. They were filming away in the hills behind Dunachton and one of the elephants got stuck in a bog and started to sink. We had to send for a breakdown truck with a crane, and they managed to haul it out and it was none the worse.

It was a great experience spending the four days with them, mixing with actors and production people from the film world, but I wouldn't change places with them for anything. They live an unreal life, entirely different from ours, and I couldn't put up with all the waiting around.

FRIDAY 26 AUGUST

I HAD ONE call this afternoon that I was not looking forward to. Canon Wheatley had called to say that his dog Sparta, which I'd been treating off and on for a while now, seemed to be getting worse every day. I feared I knew what the result of this trip would be, but there's always a hope that you'll find the animal's not as bad as you thought and there's a chance of recovery.

I pulled up outside the Canon's rectory, and Arthur was there feeding the hens which he and his wife keep on the small piece of land behind the house. I've known Arthur Wheatley, the local Episcopalian minister, for quite a few years and although I'm not really a church man I have great respect for him. He's a big, hearty chap, an ex-rugby player with thick, strong arms and biceps like a navvy's, but a gentle, warm personality. Even that morning when he must have been feeling pretty low he gave me a cheerful greeting, and his handshake was as firm as ever.

'Morning, Arthur. It's a bad job today.' On these occasions something inside you, part of your professionalism, I suppose, makes your attitude even more businesslike than usual. The only way to help the owners is to do the job as quickly and neatly as possible.

'Morning, George. You were only saying to me last week at that funeral service that you couldn't do my job. Well today I couldn't do yours, no matter what the strength of the muscles in my arms.' True enough, when I'd read a tribute to a friend at her funeral I'd been shaking like a leaf, and admired Arthur's easy way with the family, and the confidence with which he'd conducted the whole thing. Now I hoped that my own professionalism would make this experience as easy as possible for them.

We walked into the bungalow where Mrs Wheatley was waiting. She was obviously upset but was keeping it under control as so many women seem to be able to do in times of crisis. I put my small Gladstone bag down on the table.

'She's been going downhill over the last week, George.' Arthur spoke in a voice heavy with sadness as he carried the black-and-white Staffordshire bull terrier into the room.

I placed the stethoscope on the dog's chest and listened. Even though I felt pretty sure that I knew what the outcome of the examination would be I wanted to make sure that I was doing the right thing – there's no second chance at this treatment. Arthur and Mrs Wheatley looked on in tense anticipation, awaiting the verdict.

A little surprised, I took the stethoscope away. 'Her heart's not too bad – much better than I thought it would be.' I had to be careful not to give false hope, but it was definitely not as bad as I'd expected. 'Can you hold her head while I feel her tummy?'

Mrs Wheatley moved to support the dog so that I could get into a better position. Sure enough, there were the signs I'd expected to find. I knelt up. 'I'm afraid her liver's enlarged; she's getting pretty ill. There's really only one thing an owner can do for a pet in these circumstances, and that's let the dog die with dignity.'

I looked at Mrs Wheatley for confirmation that they wanted me to carry on, and received a nod; then up at Arthur's great bulk looming over us to make certain that he was in agreement. I saw his bottom lip trembling. He also nodded.

Mrs Wheatley, who seemed calm, spoke gently to her husband. 'Why don't you take the other dog out for a walk.'

With his handkerchief in one hand. Arthur shook his head, and knelt down to stroke the dog. 'She's given us so much love, George,' he whispered. 'All the children have grown up with her and they'll miss her.'

Both of them were now stroking the dog quietly, as I opened my bag and took out the syringe and the bottle containing the lethal drug. 'What we do,' I said, 'is to give her an overdose of anaesthetic and she'll just sleep away.' I don't think they were really listening to me.

'It's for the best, George, isn't it?' Arthur asked in a tone eager for reassurance.

'Oh yes, it's the last thing a caring owner can do for his pet.' I could say this with complete conviction, knowing that it was the best thing for them to do, and in many ways something I wish more owners would do before their pet really suffers.

The syringe was now loaded. I asked Mrs Wheatley to lay Sparta on a chair in the corner of the room. As she lifted her and carried her over, the Canon gently put his hand on the dog's ear.

'Which way round, George.' Mrs Wheatley's voice was strong

and almost matter of fact. I'm sure it must be her nursing training. I like to get the owners to help with their pets when they're put down. I think from a psychological point of view that it's important that they see the process through.

'Hold her with her head towards me so that I can get at a vein in her leg.' I always hope that everything will go smoothly; it's not always the easiest thing to find the vein, especially in an older dog, and I don't like it when I have to have a few goes at sticking the needle in. I clipped the hair on the leg around the vein to make it easier to locate the right spot. Without too much trouble I found the vein.

'Will you put your thumb there,' I guided Mrs Wheatley's thumb into position, 'and hold it down to make the vein rise, please.' This was the moment when I hoped everything would go as planned. I could hear a quiet sniffing from the Canon, and I didn't want to prolong the agony. The needle went in. I drew it back slightly to check that I was in the vein, and there was the telltale red in the syringe which indicated that I'd hit it first time. 'Now slacken your thumb slightly.' Mrs Wheatley did exactly as I asked and slowly I squeezed the syringe so that it released its contents.

'Good doggy, Spart,' Mrs Wheatley was constantly whispering to the dog. 'Good dog.'

'Sleepy doggy. Sleepy doggy.' The dog's eyes moved to look up at Arthur as he spoke.

The only sound from the dog was a gentle lick of its lips, almost a yawn.

'Release your thumb altogether now,' I instructed as the last of the drug left the syringe. The soothing sounds from the couple continued until the dog's eyes closed for the last time.

There was a short silence. Then Arthur spoke through his tears. 'She's gone, has she, George?'

I felt the dog's pulse. 'Oh yes. That's the old girl gone.' Inwardly I breathed a sign of relief that it had happened so smoothly. 'It's great to see how easy and painless it is for the dog, isn't it?' They both nodded, unable to speak. Now that it was over I could sense the feeling of relief in the Canon while Mrs Wheatley showed a trace of emotion for the first time. She had been so marvellous in concentrating on her role that she'd shut out her feelings. 'You'll need to give the Canon a wee dram to help his nerves,' I suggested.

Now that she'd performed her role Mrs Wheatley showed signs of the tension that she must have felt. 'I think I'll be needing one myself, George!'

'Shall I carry her out for you, Arthur?'

'Yes please, George.' Arthur stroked the dog's ear as he said this. A last farewell to a pet which had obviously meant a great deal to them both.

I walked out of the house carrying the limp form of the dog in my arms. The sun was streaming through the trees, and brought a sense of relief to me. I laid Sparta on the back seat of the car, covered her with a sheet and shut the door.

The Canon and Mrs Wheatley walked slowly down the drive, Arthur carrying a small grey parcel. 'A small thank you, George.'

I read the label. 'Free range eggs from Canon Wheatley's hens.' I laughed. 'Do they come with a blessing on them?'

'No. The blessing goes on you, not on the eggs, George.' Arthur replied with some of his big grin in evidence again now.

'Well, that's great. Thanks very much.' I shook hands with him. Mrs Wheatley passed me my bag, which I put in the car and slammed the boot. I turned back to her. 'You were great. I'll give you a job as a veterinary nurse any day.'

She laughed shakily as I gave her a big hug. 'Thanks, George.'

I drove away, leaving them standing by their gate. I've done this job hundreds of times over the years, but it doesn't get any easier no matter how many times you've done it.

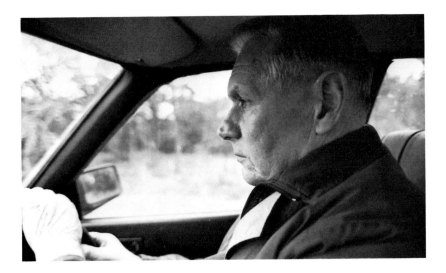

SUNDAY 4 SEPTEMBER

T HE ARRIVAL OF a new assistant is always an interesting occasion, especially when it's a person I haven't even met. That was the case with the latest of my assistants, Neil Cockburn, who turned up today.

Willie and I had been very busy in the practice and I decided that it was about time we had a third pair of hands again – someone who could help out with the routine work at first and then move on to other areas after a while.

I was very careful about the wording of the advert. I didn't want to attract the wrong kind of person. A lot of people have too romantic an idea of what life up here is going to be like. In fact it can be very tough, and it's often hard to see any glamour in it at all.

I advertised in the *Veterinary Record* and we had quite a few replies, from all over, even one from Canada. A couple of applicants came up for interviews, but they weren't suitable. We were busy and I got fed up with all that fuss, so in the end I appointed Neil Cockburn over the phone. Although it was only a brief conversation, he sounded a nice kind of chap. I've taken on people in this way before, and not been wrong so far.

Neil is a graduate from Cambridge so he'll probably be kind of posh! I was at university with one of his professors, who spoke of him in glowing terms when I phoned for a reference. He's also got a good Scots surname, Cockburn, even if he is an Englishman living in Wales at the moment. It does mean that now I'll be outnumbered three to one in the practice, with Willie and Jane being incomers as well, but it takes a lot to keep a good Scotsman down!

We've had a real mixture of assistants here over the years, some good and others not. It's not always the veterinary side of the work that causes problems.

There was one assistant quite a few years ago who became known as 'Crashing Kate'. She was a blooming expensive thing to have about the place. In ten months she damaged the car five times. From what I hear she's still crashing cars now!

Then again some of them don't really get on with animals. They give off some sort of odour when they approach an animal which upsets and frightens them, and that makes it difficult for everyone. You always hope that your new assistant will have an empathy with the animals. The best one we ever had was a chap called Cora. He could handle animals really well; he was in tune with them – in fact I think there might have been something kind of animal about him. The girls around the district thought so too!

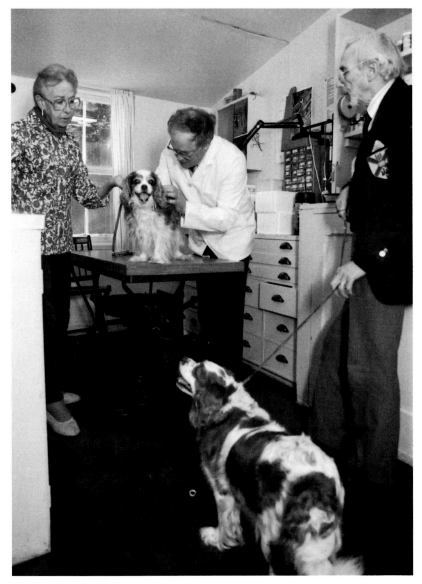

Willie at work in the surgery.

Sadly for the profession he left his wife, trotted off to America and became a Buddhist monk.

On the whole, though, I've been very lucky with my assistants. Willie came to the practice about sixteen years ago and now he's a respected member of the community. We get on pretty well on the whole, although he's given in his notice three times. I suppose it's a bit like a marriage, really: you have your good and bad days, and your ups and downs.

It was a coincidence that brought Willie to Grantown in the first place. My assistant at the time was leaving and everyone in the district knew that. News tends to travel up here! A Mrs Boyd who had moved to Tomatin from Derbyshire phoned me to say that her doctor back home had a son who was a vet. She said she'd heard that he wasn't very happy where he was, and was looking for a new job. So I wrote to one Willie Hollick, and he came up initially for a few months, and stayed. It wasn't long before he met a local girl, Helen, who lived in Nethybridge, and married her, and of course, once you marry a Highland girl you're stuck up here! Willie's the kind of person you've got to get to know, and once you do, you realise that he's a genuine kind of chap. He's hard-working, great with the large animals, and especially good at blood testing – he can get blood out of a stone. He's fitted in very well and the clients like him. I hope the new boy will be like that.

Most people who go to veterinary college these days have a real fondness for animals, and if you're fond of animals you're halfway there. When the animal you're dealing with bites or kicks you, it's not really very easy to keep your cool if you don't have any feeling for it in the first place! My liking for and interest in animals came when I was a youngster. In my early teens we lived on the periphery of Glasgow and there was a farm right opposite. I used to wander over and help with the animals occasionally and I suppose I just got fond of them and sort of drifted into being a vet because of that contact.

If Neil's as good as I'm told he is then we'll be fine. He shouldn't have any trouble with the physical side of the work anyway. He looks a big hearty kind of chap, and he's just been on holiday climbing in the Alps, so he must be tough.

Waiting for Neil to arrive this afternoon I couldn't help thinking about my own student days. I'm sure they were different from Neil's in some ways and very similar in others.

I started college in 1943 at the age of seventeen during some of the darkest days of the war. My brother was training to be a pilot in the RAF. I can remember him coming home with his wings on his tunic, and I really envied him for achieving such status. I regret not having been in the services; I'm sure it's the only place you get such a strong feeling of camaraderie. It wasn't to be, though – I was too young, so I carried on with my studying.

I went to one of the two veterinary colleges in Edinburgh, the Royal Dick, named after William Dick who founded it. Edinburgh was a great place for us to get our education and learn the ways of the world. At least fifty per cent of my fellow students were English and they were much more sophisticated than us Scots. This was partly due to the fact that they were nearly all one or two years older than us. At that age a couple of extra years meant that they'd seen a lot more of life than we Scots lads who'd all been at local schools and never been away from home much.

I must admit my horizons needed widening; I was very, very raw. When I arrived in Edinburgh I was just a country boy landing in the big city. The Royal Dick was not then part of the university, only affiliated to it, so there were no places in halls of residence for us and I went into digs. Living in someone else's home was a strange experience for me.

If I was raw there were others who were even more unworldly. One was a chap called Bill Corrigal, who I became friendly with. We have remained friends ever since.

After we'd been in Edinburgh a couple of weeks Bill decided that he wanted to buy a new hat. So we went down to Princes Street and went to the poshest shop, which was Forsyth's. As we approached the huge doors a commissionaire in a frock coat swung them open for us. We walked in, trying to look as though we'd done this sort of thing every day of our lives. He asked us which department we wanted. Determined not to be intimidated, Corrigal stood tall and said in a confident voice, 'We want a bonnet.'

The commissionaire looked at him and in that way of people who think they're superior said, '*Hats* are on the third floor, sir.' He didn't even attempt to hide his contempt for these two country bumpkins.

We found a great selection of bonnets which Bill proceeded to try on. Eventually a decision was made and, in a rather grand way for a young chap, Bill summoned an assistant across and asked the price. She told us, and his confident air took a dive. It was as much as we'd have expected to pay for a whole outfit. So we left without the bonnet and with our tails between our legs. The commissionaire must have seen others leave in the same way over the years, and seemed to take great pleasure in asking, 'Did Sir find what he required?' Bill mumbled something about 'not the right colour' and we left as quickly as we could.

With the war being on, the Dick College had a battalion of the Home Guard. We all had to turn out for parades, and were issued with army rifles, uniform and the rest of the kit. I can remember that in 1944 at the time of the invasion we were all stood by in case we were needed. I think if we had been drafted in to help out we'd have gone willingly and keenly. We were pretty fit in those days, but God help the regular forces if we had been called upon to do our duty. Our ideas of fighting a modern battle were pretty dim indeed.

We used to go on night exercises in a park near Holyrood Palace. It was just far enough away from the city for us to be left alone. Almost. We used to have one battalion, and the dental students another. We had to try and penetrate their lines, which involved creeping through the gorse bushes. The manoeuvres were quite often held on Saturday nights, and it was common to hear a volley of abusive language coming from a gorse bush a few hundred feet away from where you were crawling along, and then the sound of fighting breaking out. It was rarely between the two sides taking part in the exercise, but more likely between a budding Casanova and an unlucky soldier who'd happened across a courting couple hidden in the bushes. Although flushing out amorous couples wasn't the intended object of the exercise, it added a certain spice to the events.

Like all students past and present we were always hard up for money. Because I had a Carnegie scholarship, I was better off than many of my peers, but we were all still for ever trying to find new ways to earn some extra cash. During term time there was easy money to be had working as coupon checkers at a football pools company in Edinburgh called Strangs.

It was a pretty sordid sort of place with all the windows blacked out, making it dim and dingy inside. There was a huge room with nothing but long tables and chairs and rows of people sitting there. You weren't allowed to speak to the person next to you – if you did you were out. The coupons arrived with all manner of things on them, very often bits of egg or jam, or worse.

When you came across a winning coupon you just put it into your top pocket so that it stuck out, and there were people circulating who would pick them up. This was all done without a word being spoken. The whole place was run in absolute silence – the only sound would be the constant rustle of the coupons being turned over. It was almost Dickensian.

I must have marked thousands and thousands of coupons there and I never saw more than a third dividend, so I think from that your chances of winning were pretty remote. But the wages were good: £2.50 for Saturday, and £4 for Sunday. Quite often if they were busy there'd be checking to be done on a Monday as well. No one asked for any identification, even though during the war everyone had ID cards, and at the end of the day it was cash in hand.

Mind you, I'd earned it by the end of a weekend spent locked away inside. I don't think it helped in the study of veterinary matters because you were spending time away from studying, making money, and then when you had the cash you just went out and wasted more time spending it.

I discovered that during the holidays there was another way to earn good cash, and that was in the docks. I spent my vacations there between 1943 and 1945. The pay as a docker was something like £2 a day at a time when the average wage must have been about £3 a week. I was lucky that an uncle of mine was in charge of part of the docks in Glasgow and he used to arrange that I was taken on.

The full-time licensed dockers were a real closed shop you virtually had to be born into, but when they needed extra dockers they called upon the casual labour squad. For this you queued up on the quayside, and as long as you weren't recognised as a trouble-maker you were taken on. Uncle had also tipped the clerk off to make sure I got on the list.

It was quite easy work, starting at seven o'clock in the morning, after travelling by tramcar to the docks. They were a real mixed bunch. Like the pools company, nobody asked for identification when you signed on, and again it was cash in hand. I reckon a good sixty per cent of the squad were people on the run from one thing or another. There were deserters, men hiding from the police, Irishmen with very dubious pasts who'd come across in search of work, and me, a seventeen-year-old innocent from the sticks. I got on pretty well with them, but I had to be careful. They hated my Uncle George who ran the docks. They'd see him walking around in his soft hat and say, 'There's that bastard,' with amazing venom. He'd pass by and never look at me. We both knew that if he'd shown any recognition, and they'd discovered who I was, they'd have thrown me in the docks. I'd often glance down into the water, filthy black oily-looking stuff with all sorts of scum and dirt floating on the surface, and then look at the hard bunch of crooks I was working with, and join in heartily with the abuse!

The money we earned in these varied ways helped towards making our social life more interesting – these were the days when phrases like 'going Dutch' hadn't even been thought of. Every Saturday night there was a dance, and our partners were as often as not from the nearby Domestic Science College, or the Dough School as it was called. The girls lived in Atholl Crescent, closely supervised and protected by their matron from the intentions, amorous or innocent, of the boys from the Dick Vet college which was temptingly close by. The house rules, known intimately by all vet students, were that the girls had to be in by eleven o'clock sharp at night. It must have been quite a sight on a Saturday night, the railings in Atholl Crescent outside the Dough School, lined with girls and their aspiring veterinary surgeon boyfriends. As soon as eleven o'clock came, they'd vanish as one, even if they'd been in mid-embrace. Latecomers had to knock on the door and the matron would demand to know where they'd been, who with and what they'd been up to.

Despite all the obstacles put in their way, some of them were known to transgress from time to time. I don't think I ought to dwell too much on the details of those occasions, suffice to say that more than once a bit of clambering through open windows on the first floor was required.

So our Saturday nights fell into a regular pattern: five to eight o'clock at the football coupon firm, Strangs, then to our favourite pub 'The Southern' where we used to drink beer, not whisky in those days. It didn't take many beers to get us merry, so when we had got steamed up, we went around to the dance in the college with all these lovely young ladies. There were never any fights at the dances, because there were never any gate crashers. All the lads knew each other, even though the students in the final year were exalted people who we used to see going around and didn't presume to talk to. We had a good deterrent to gate crashers, vet bouncers. Out of all the two hundred or so students at the Dick Vet College I was one of the smallest, and that made for good quality strongmen on the door.

Our student days weren't all about making money and enjoying ourselves – we did attend some lectures from time to time. One of the lecturers was a Colonel Buchanan-Smith who later became Lord Balerno. He was a big imposing chap with a very military bearing, and he used to march into the room and start lecturing, machine-gun fashion. This was before the days of slides and there was an epidiascope for illustrations. You put a photograph in the bottom of the machine and it would project it on to a screen. We were in one of these lectures one day, with the room in darkness. The colonel was going on, and the photographs to do with genetics were flashing up on to the screen, when all of a sudden a picture of a nude female appeared. I really thought the colonel was going to explode. One of the students had slipped in before the lecture and added it to the pile of illustrations waiting to be shown. To give the colonel his due he saw the joke and I'm sure he became less formal after that experience. I never discovered if he gave the photograph back to the student.

Meat inspection was and is a subject which is taken very seriously in Scotland. It's part of our veterinary duties, so it's taught in detail and with precision at university. We used to have to go out to the city's slaughter-house once a week at about half past five in the morning, and the lecturer in charge would show us how to look for disease in carcasses and so on. The slaughter-men were a tough crowd of big, strong, brusque men, always caked in blood, rushing around with their long knives hanging about their waists. But there was one little thickset chap who would always stop and talk to us. He had discovered that there was easy money to be made from us. If you gave him a shilling he would fill a jam jar with the warm blood from the jugular vein of a newly slaughtered animal and drink it down. This was a great treat for us to watch.

One of the other lecturers at the college, Johnny Burgess, was an eminent surgeon, much admired and respected in the college and throughout the profession. He was a quiet, unassuming man but was renowned as a surgeon throughout the whole of Scotland. In the days before antibiotics and all the modern treatments we have now, he used to get remarkable surgical results. When he was operating Johnny used to smoke a cigarette nearly all the time, and the ash from the cigarette used quite often to drop off into the wound. I've often wondered if that was part of the secret of his success.

When we got into the final year or even towards the end of the fourth year we were offered the chance to do locums. In that way most of us were better off than the young chaps who come out of college today. It was less of a strain when we actually started in practice because most of us had done quite a bit of unofficial work by then. When I was a student an awful lot of veterinary surgeons were on their own in practice, so if they took ill or went away for any reason they had to get a locum. If they couldn't get a qualified vet then it was quite common for them to phone up the college and speak to Johnny Burgess who would come along with his cigarette hanging out of the corner of his mouth and ask if we'd like to go and look after such and such a place for a week. This was strictly against the rules of the Royal College, but it went on. I think things were a bit more free and easy then, and the farmers were easier to please.

If we had a choice of locum work we'd opt for somewhere far away from Scotland in a place where we wouldn't be known, so that if anything went wrong we hoped we wouldn't be found out.

I DID A locum in 1946 at Honiton in Devon. A friend of mine who was newly qualified was in practice there and his boss was away, so I filled in. The only instruction I was given was that if I went to a calving case and the calf was dead I was to take the carcass back for the vet's wife who kept boxer dogs. I didn't agree with this arrangement, but being the new boy, kept quiet about it. It wasn't long before I was sent to a cow which had given birth to a dead calf, and the farmer, knowing the arrangement with the vet, put the body in a bag and presented it to me to put in my car. I was driving a two-seater Austin with a dicky seat at the back which my unwelcome passenger took. I had other calls to make and I didn't fancy taking the body around with me, so I stopped in a quiet place, threw the calf over a wall and drove off.

I finished the locum and returned to college. One day I was engrossed in a lecture when the formal figure of Joe People, the college janitor, entered the room. He was in his usual attire of frock coat, with his full complement of medals jangling on his chest. I was summoned to see the principal of the college, Sir Arthur Oliver, a formidable ex-Indian Army officer. He sat there very aloof, looking at me with great disdain, and informed me that a policeman was waiting to interview me about an alleged offence in Honiton.

For once I was at a loss to think of any illegal act I'd committed while in Devon. Rather than allaying any fears which the situation gave rise to, that only served to make me even more apprehensive about what I was about to be confronted with. The janitor was obviously enjoying all this as he frogmarched me to a side room where a police sergeant was waiting.

As I walked in he rose. 'Mr Rafferty?'

I gulped yes, and he continued in a formal voice. 'I am here to charge you with an offence against public health.'

The janitor's expression was that of a small child about to be given a great treat, but it turned to disappointment as the sergeant asked him to leave us alone. When the door had closed he explained what lay behind the charge. The water supply to a village near Honiton had been contaminated because a dead calf had been dumped in a stream which fed the village. The calf had been traced back to the farmer who told the police that he'd given it to a certain Scottish vet who'd been doing a locum. I thought that there was nothing for it but to tell the truth, and explain that although I had technically been responsible for this mis-demeanour I felt that it was a bit harsh to be charged with such a serious offence.

Having listened to my story the policeman sat back in his chair and thought for a moment. 'Now,' he said, 'if you plead not guilty you'll have to travel down to Devon to stand trial.' My heart sank at the thought of a cross-examination, and having to explain my motives during what was in any case an illegal locum. 'On the other hand,' suggested the sergeant, 'Might it have hap-pened this way. . . .'

He went on to explain that perhaps I'd been given the calf to dispose of, and had returned to the surgery to find that the dicky seat was empty and the corpse gone. I then retraced my steps but was unable to find any sign of the body. So I assumed that someone had found it and buried it.

Having listened to the sergeant's version of the sequence of events, it was strange how instantly I remembered that this was in fact a true representation of the circumstances on the day in question. I was relieved when the charges were dropped, and I was a free man to pursue my career.

For the rest of my days at the Dick Vet college I was always a marked men in Sir Arthur's eyes, but ever since that incident I've always found officers of the law very friendly.

So by the time I qualified I'd done quite a few locums. When Neil starts with us this week he's bound to find it harder than I did because he just won't have had the experience. We've got to break him in gently because they all come out of college greener than the grass these days, and it's our duty to help him get to know the way of things. When they have had to treat something there's usually been someone standing over them checking what they're doing. Then when they come out into the real world they're on their own all of a sudden. They're sent off in their car with a lot of drugs and maybe presented with a valuable animal and it's all theirs to deal with. There's no one to turn around to and ask, 'What should I do?'

We've all been in that situation at one time, though. I can remember running to the car to look up a textbook to check the symptoms. Mind you, I can't think of a better bunch of clients to throw him to for his first experience. They're real kindly folk and they'll know that he's newly qualified and pretty wet behind the ears, so they'll try to put him at his ease, unlike some other parts of the country where I'm sure just the opposite would be true.

It's often not the veterinary side of things which the young lads find most difficult, but the business aspect of the job. Most of them will not have been in a situation where they've had to deal with money, and sometimes the most difficult part to get used to is asking for the £5 or whatever for treating an animal. But I worked for a great chap in Hampshire who used to say, 'Never mind asking for your fee, you're only asking for your own.' And I suppose he's right; we've nothing else to sell other than our skill and when we've given advice why shouldn't we ask for a fee.

At five o'clock the doorbell went. Jane was just finishing off preparing the tea. She'd decided that we should have some local Spey salmon as an introduction to the delights of the area. I opened the door to reveal a tall, blond, good-looking young lad, who I guessed straight away must be Neil.

'Hello. Mr Rafferty?' he asked in a slightly nervous way.

'Hello, Neil. Welcome to Grantown.' In the drive was an estate car piled high with cases and books. I could recognise some of the textbooks even from a distance! 'Get your father: we've got tea ready for you both.'

I CUT ANOTHER slice of bread. 'We've got marvellous bread here, made by Walker's of Aberlour.' I had to introduce Neil to the joys of local produce. As the meal continued the conversation became easier.

Neil was obviously nervous, but a great deal less so than most young men in his position. 'You've had new graduates here before, haven't you?'

'Yes, you can see my grey hair, can't you?' They all laughed, but there was an element of truth in it.

After tea Jane showed Neil around his new home. He gets a bungalow just around the corner from us which I bought for use by our assistants. It means that he's close enough to get to the surgery quickly, but not so close that it feels as if we're keeping an eye on him. I wouldn't like to think too much about some of the things which I imagine have gone on in the house over the years, but there's that expression about what the eye doesn't see the heart doesn't grieve over, or in this case worry about or even get jealous about!

WHEN NEIL HAD unloaded his possessions from his father's car, he came over to the house for a brief fireside chat. I like to welcome them into the profession when it's their first job; after all, it's a big day for them. We raised our glasses, toasted veterinary surgeons, and I gave him my 'introductory speech'.

'The veterinary profession', I said to him, 'is one of the last of the caring professions which isn't owned by national or local government, and that puts a terrific pressure on us. We've got the welfare of our patients to think of, the economic position of our clients to consider, but at the end of the day we've got to make a living for ourselves!'

Neil sat on the settee with his glass of whisky listening intently to all this. I hope I didn't sound too self-important!

'You'll find that we're very cost-conscious here,' I went on. 'Unfortunately we don't live in the stockbroker belt for small animals, so most of our income is from the large animals, and we have to remember that it's our business to keep the farmers in business.'

I think all this was at the forefront of my mind because only the day before young Gertie had come into the surgery for advice. Her family farms sheep at Calier in the Braes of Glenlivet. They've had three die in recent days from acute Pasteurellosis, a germ which causes sudden death. She turned up this time with one of them in the back of her estate car. We pulled it out and I took it into the garage where we quite often do post mortems on animals if we're unsure of the cause of death. In this case when we opened it up it looked like sure signs of the disease again.

Gertie was then faced with a terrible choice. Should she inject the whole flock of four hundred against it, which would cost over £200, or leave it in the hope that only a few more might die. There she was, a girl in her mid-twenties, having to make decisions like that. All I could do was to put the options to her and tell her what I thought she should do, but it wasn't my livelihood that would be affected if the decision was wrong. I suppose if we injected she'd be certain that they'd be safe, but would never know whether it had been the right decision or not. Of course if we left them and many more of them died she'd have to live with the wrong choice for a long time. When you're talking about a farm which may have a monthly income of just a few hundred pounds, a couple of sheep worth maybe a hundred pounds each could tip the balance too far. She decided to wait and see what happened.

'We have a lot of valuable cattle up here,' I continued to Neil. 'A lot of Smithfield champions have been bred in the district. A champion can be a valuable asset to a farm, and it means that we really have to get our treatment right. The feed manufacturers all come knocking offering the farmers financial inducements to endorse their product. The standard of stockmanship is very high up here because it's handed down through the generations, from father to son. Have you much experience of cattle, Neil?'

Neil had been listening intently to my diatribe for all this time. 'Well, only what I've done in practice, really,' he replied. 'Obviously, coming from a town background, I have to place myself on a very different level from these farmers who've been doing it all their lives.'

Time to sound a small warning note. 'But remember you're the expert.' I have great respect for the farmers, but you've got to teach new graduates that they must command respect from the farmers as well, or else they'll never be trusted.

'I've bought you a new car to start your career in.' I was glad to see Neil look surprised at this news. 'It's only done about fifty

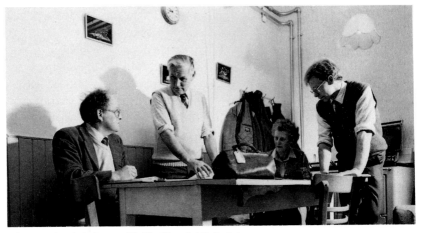

The morning briefing on Neil's (far right) first day.

miles, so you'll have to look after it and keep it clean. You start off with sixty per cent no claims bonus and we expect it to stay that way, so don't go driving stupidly!'

I'd bought him a new Ford Fiesta. They're front wheel drive and pretty good in the icy weather. 'You'll find that in the winter I'll give you plenty of reminders about the ice, and about driving carefully! And one important thing, when you go into a farmyard, always turn the car facing out before you park – for a quick getaway in case you kill anything!' I could see that Neil was unsure whether to take this piece of advice seriously or not, but it really *was* quite serious. Bitter experience has taught me that there's nothing worse than a lot of manoeuvring about in the car to get away if you've been unsuccessful on your call! 'And don't park near a tractor or animals because either can do a lot of damage to a modern car. They're a bit like tin cans – one shove from a cow's hoof and the whole panel's gone.'

The lecture over, Neil went back to spend his first night in his new abode, and I settled down to write up today's visits in our diary. It's a record of the treatment given to every animal we see, and it means that if one of the others makes a return visit we'll know what's been done before. I left it out ready to show Neil in the morning. He's got to start somewhere, and it's important for any new member of the team to get on top of the basics as soon as possible. They can then concentrate on the veterinary side of the business, and not worry about the routine.

Tomorrow will be his first day.

MONDAY 5 SEPTEMBER

NEIL'S FIRST DAY out in the practice. I had a few interesting cases planned for that morning, so he was to spend it with me. The door-bell rang at 8.15AM and when I opened it there he was in his brand new outfit and wellington boots, carrying one of his textbooks with him.

Neil's introduction to the practice was to be with Jimmy Forbes, who breeds Smithfield champion cattle. In a strange sort of way I was really quite proud to be able to show off one of our top class farmers to this new graduate. Jimmy's telephone message had said that he had a cow with milk fever. Most of the farmers are so experienced that they have a pretty good idea of what's wrong with their animals before they phone us.

We packed the car and drove to the farm which is just outside Grantown.

'Morning, Jimmy. This is my new young man, Neil Cockburn.' Jimmy's a fairly short chap with dark complexion and rough skin which has been hardened by years of exposure to the wind and rain. He looked pretty tired. I'll give him the benefit of the doubt and say that it was because he'd been up all night calving, though I'm sure he'd not be as generous to me!

'She calved yesterday, and went down this morning, George.' In front of us the black-and-white Friesian cow was lying still in the hay. Milk fever is caused by the cow's blood calcium going down after calving and we do a simple replacement therapy by putting a calcium drip into her to bring it back to normal.

'You check her temperature, Neil, and we'll see if Jimmy's diagnosis is right.'

'It's not often wrong, George!' replied Jimmy, which is true.

I'd prepared the bottle and the special flutter valve while we'd been talking and I had to hit the vein now. 'I always get nervous when I've got a young assistant watching me trying to hit a vein!' I could see that Neil wasn't sure whether I was joking or not. I got the needle in to the vein first time.

'You were obviously out playing darts last night, George,' said Jimmy in a mock congratulatory way.

I told Neil to hold the bottle up high. 'We're in a hurry, Neil, and Jimmy's just as impatient as ourselves.' We chatted on as the liquid ran into the cow's vein. If you're lucky the cow some-times gets up as soon as it's all run in. I think it depends on the psychology of the particular animal: with active, aggressive cows they're up and off, straight away, whereas if they're sort of placid they're inclined to lie for a wee while.

Jimmy stroked the cow's head absentmindedly as we watched the calcium level in the bottle go down. 'Did you enjoy the show, George?' he asked. It had been the annual Grantown Show a couple of weeks before, the social highlight of the farming year.

'Aye, it was great. I only had two things to attend to. A calf which sort of went mad, and a wee lassie with a mouse with a lump on it. She'd entered it into the pets' parade – I think really just as an excuse for some free veterinary advice.'

Neil laughed. I'm not sure how much they teach you about dealing with the human side of things at college these days.

'That's the lot.' Neil took the bottle down as he spoke. And with a gentle nudge the cow was up and walking.

'The doctors can't produce a cure like that!' I said to Neil with great satisfaction. It's always good when your treatment is successful with the new boy watching.

NEXT ON THE list, some medicine to drop off in Tomintoul, the second highest village in Scotland. It was for a farmer whose real name is George Irvine, but who is known universally as 'Wee Dod'. Because a lot of our clients live some distance away we often leave medicines at a suitable halfway point for them to pick up. I was leaving this one with Ella, Wee Dod's sister.

As we drove up the main street I thought of a vital piece of information to pass on to Neil. 'You've got to watch your speed in Tomintoul. There's very often a speed trap here.' Neil looked quite understandably bemused. It's a small town with one long main street and hardly the place you'd expect to find a radar trap.

We pulled up at Ella's house, and I rang the doorbell. The door opened, revealing a short, grey-haired woman.

'Ella, I've brought the penicillin for Wee Dod.'

'Uh huh,' she took the parcel.

'And how are you today?'

'Just terrible, George. My legs are playing up again, the knees have gone.'

'You'll have to come over and see me!'

'Not likely. I know you too well – you'll take them off!'

BACK IN THE car, we passed the road which leads to the Braes of Glenlivet. It's an unusual area in that many of the farmers who live there are Roman Catholics. They're not incomers either; they've been there for generations. We were originally all Roman Catholics up here but then John Knox came around and started the Reformation and turned us all into protestants. His disciples travelled all over the countryside converting people, but they missed remote places like the Braes of Glenlivet, which I suppose gives an indication of how remote some of these areas are. The same sort of thing happened in the Western Isles in places like Barra: wherever John Knox's men failed to reach they retained their old religion. Not that it makes any difference! It just reminded me to fill Neil in on the local idiosyncracies.

A lot of the folk in Glenlivet are related. One of the farmers over there is an incomer – he's only been living there for about fifty years. We were talking the other day about this and he said, 'If you kick somebody's backside at Ballindalloch it dirls all the way to Tomintoul.' If you hit your hand with a hammer it 'dirls'. In other words if you upset somebody at one end of the family chain the repercussions go all the way to the other. It's true. I've known people I hadn't seen for ages who would make their displeasure clear, and I'd be trying to work out what I'd said or done; then later I'd find that some time previously I'd shouted at their cousin twenty miles away. So you have to be careful what you say.

OUR NEXT VISIT gave me the chance to talk to Neil about one of the most useful, oft-used and indeed my favourite medicines, whisky. We had a call to The Glenlivet distillery where I had some Highland cows to test for tuberculosis, and also to try and persuade the manager to take part in a new Highland health scheme for sheep. I explained to Neil how important whisky is to the district, not only to those of us who drink it, but also as a source of employment. The Glenlivet distillery is quite an old one, I think it was one of the first ones to register under the Act of Parliament early in the nineteenth century which required distilleries to pay excise duty. There are lots of stories of people back then putting the whisky into casks and taking it across the hills down to the Lowlands, and selling it there to avoid the excisemen.

There used to be an exciseman in each distillery who had the keys for the warehouse, and no one was allowed in unless he was there. The by-products of the distilling process – what's left of the barley and malt after the alcohol's been taken out – are a very valuable first class cattle feed. If the distilleries went into recession it would affect the farming community badly for that reason, as well as the fact that they pay good wages to their workers. So I always think that the more whisky we drink the more good we're doing the farming community.

The drams you used to get after calving cases in Glenlivet were something to look forward to. They had usually been obtained shall we say 'surreptitiously' from a distillery by one of the sons of the farm or a relative or neighbour who worked there. You always knew you were in for a good quality dram when a plain bottle appeared, with no label. Sometimes it would be an old lemonade bottle or for some reason it often seemed to be a Drambuie bottle. If they were taking a wee drop home just to have for themselves, they certainly weren't going to take immature raw stuff: it was always the finest fifteen- or twenty-year-old stuff out of a cask in a bonded warehouse. So you could always be sure that whisky after a calving case in Glenlivet or Tomintoul was the very best.

One thing you had to be careful about was the stuff that came out of the unlabelled bottles was very much stronger than the whisky you buy in a shop. Some of it was over 100 degrees proof. If you had one small glass of it you certainly knew you'd had a dram, and it was no good having another if you were driving.

When we arrived at The Glenlivet distillery, Accie Christie the herdsman had the animals in the barn ready for us. The Highland cattle are quite fearsome to look at with their long, shaggy brown coats, and huge horns. They're not really dangerous, but they can give you quite a jab with their horns if they happen to turn at the wrong moment, so you have to exercise a bit of caution working with them. There aren't many people with folds of Highland cattle these days – the distillery keeps them mainly for the image and the tourists. They are fetching good money abroad, though, so maybe they'll come back into fashion.

We saw the stots, which I explained to Neil are castrated male animals, what would be called bullocks in England, and took some samples from the cows. Then we went into the distillery manager's office where inevitably we were offered a wee dram as we discussed the new sheep scheme. I asked if I could take mine home in a bottle since I was driving, and he obliged by producing a miniature. I explained the idea behind the scheme was that if the sheep were blood tested and proved clear of disease, their owners would be able to sell them for a higher price. We get problems up here with enzootic abortions where the ewes abort their lambs because of a disease. The tests I was proposing would establish that the flock was clear.

I managed to persuade him to join the scheme which by coincidence is being run by an old assistant of mine, Harry Ross, who's now one of the area's chief veterinary research officers. It'll mean more work for us, and I'm always pleased to drum up new business.

LAST ON OUR list today was a visit to Madgie McQueen's croft on the other side of town to castrate, or 'cut' as we call it, some of her bull calves. The croft is set in a valley which is incredibly beautiful in its ruggedness and wildness, and Madgie keeps a few horses and a few cattle and scrapes a living from the land. It must be a pretty hard way to earn a crust.

When we turned up Madgie was waiting for us. I introduced Neil and we started to put our boots and overtrousers on. 'I've got a hole in my boots, George.' Madgie's face had a big grin on it. Her polished, rounded cheeks, large bosom and strong body shook as she laughed.

'I've got a hole as well, Madgie. We're both too mean to buy new ones.'

Hugh joined us. He lives at the croft next door, and is usually around to help out whenever needed. They're both about the same height, with broad faces that have seen years of hard work in the open air. 'Madgie's a very important person in the district, Neil,' I said. 'Next year she's going to be the president of the Strathspey Farmers' Club.' Madgie laughed and again her whole body shook.

We went into the byre, where half-a-dozen calves were waiting for us. 'Working in a croft you don't have many facilities,' I explained to Neil.

'No mod cons here, George,' agreed Madgie.

In the far end of the barn Hugh had rigged up an old gate to run the cattle behind, and use as a holding pen, from which we could take them out one by one. 'Have you got a halter, Hugh?' I asked.

He produced a great length of something which looked

unusual. 'That's made from an old parachute harness, George,' explained Madgie. 'It's pretty strong.' I didn't like to ask Madgie where she got the parachute from in the first place.

'It's all to be stots in here, is it, Madgie?' I asked, and she confirmed the instructions. I roped the first animal, and Hugh opened the gate to allow it through.

The next thing I knew I was running down the length of the barn being taken for a jog by the animal. I couldn't really see, but I think there was a suggestion of a smile on Neil's face. The calf really didn't want to be tied up. Perhaps it knew what was in store for it. As if to make a final bid for freedom it shook the halter off and and ran back up the other end. 'It's too big,' I said. 'I'll have to get my own halter from the car, Madgie.'

I brought it back in. 'I made this halter myself. You have to be a university graduate to use it.' I saw Neil looking at me.

We tied the first one up and started work on it. We castrate the males because in that way males and females can be kept together. If we didn't they'd forever be serving the females. As we went along I explained to Neil the way I like to go about the job. 'We inject about 5 c.cs of anaesthetic into the top of each testicle.'

The animal jumped about as I injected it. It wasn't so much the injection – we use a very fine needle – but the fact that it didn't like being held. In a bigger farm we'd put them into a cattle crate, but here Hugh had the halter tied to an upright in the byre, while Madgie used her body to wedge the animal against the stall. 'I like to use the old-fashioned Jeyes Fluid to disinfect the scrotum, Neil, You can work with it day in day out and it never affects your hands like a lot of the surgical scrubs do. Some of them seem to take the fat out of your hands and you get dermatitis, but I think there must be tar in this stuff. We buy it in 5-gallon drums because we use so much of it.'

I went on to show in detail how I like to cut the scrotum and pull the testicle out. 'We just use the scalpel blade without the handle, because if the animal kicks it won't hit the handle and drive the blade up into itself.' Neil was bent over, watching with great concentration what was going on. I could see him lapping up the instructions as we went along.

IT REMINDED ME of the first time I took Willie out. He'd been qualified just over a year. We went to cut some calves, and I

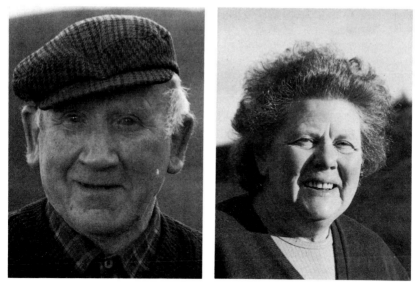

Hugh and Madgie

showed him how to do it, as I had Neil today. Then I got him to do one. He started on it and I said, 'No, if you hold it that way you'll cut yourself.'

'Oh, I prefer to do it this way,' he replied confidently. So I said nothing more. The next time he was sent out on his own to castrate some cattle I got a message from the hospital to say that he was there having stitches put in. I think he's changed his method since then.

After I'd done one I let Neil have a go. It's always more difficult to do a job with the boss standing over you, but he seemed to be doing really well. He took a long time, but then I suppose that's something that will improve with experience.

Hugh and Madgie looked on as he worked, Hugh had a big grin on his face. He's seen many of my assistants do this job, and I'm sure it added a bit of interest to the whole thing for him today, to watch how the latest one got on. 'You be careful not to cut too deep, Neil,' I said. 'Farmers don't like to see blood!'

Madgie and Hugh laughed. I've had men out watching me do this job who've virtually got their legs crossed as they watch. I always explain to them that it's all in their mind. The calves have had a local anaesthetic, so they won't feel a thing. They don't think about their sexual prowess like humans do, and they're too young to know anyway.

Neil finished the job, with only a bit of tussle with the second testicle. In just a few hours it's difficult to judge him fully, but from what I've seen I think he's going to be 'an ornament to the profession', as we used to say.

We all went into the farmhouse for tea and cake. 'You've got to remember not to stay too long having tea, Neil,' I told him as we walked inside. 'Our clients are too polite to tell us to get out, and you have to remember that they've got work to do and so have we. We haven't got time to sit around chatting all day.'

Madgie and Hugh were smiling at my instructions to Neil. 'I've never known you to feel the urge to rush away, George, when a drop of the hard stuff is on offer anyway!' Hugh gave Neil a wink as he said this. Neil looked around him at the paintings on the walls, not hanging but actually painted on the walls. Madgie does all of them, miniature murals, scenes of farm life.

Eventually we left, having stayed longer than I would have done normally, but it was good for Neil to meet some of our clients on his first day. I'm sure the hospitality everywhere was a pleasant surprise to him, if nothing else.

ON THE WAY back home I asked Neil what he thought of the practice from his brief introduction. He seemed to be impressed with the variety of work and I suppose that's true. I think you'd be hard pressed to find a better bunch than the farmers up here. They know their business inside out and they're entertaining and hospitable with it. I told Neil to remember that some of them are getting on a bit now and you have to help them if there are cattle to be caught. It keeps you fit anyway. I often come away from a farm and think to myself, that person I told to catch a cow or pull the gate or shouted to hold on to the rope tighter was over seventy, and you know they never complain. They've done it all their lives, I suppose. I only hope I'll be as lively as they are when I get into my next decade.

NEIL WILL SPEND the next few days with either Willie or me, learning the ropes. It will be interesting to see how he develops. It's too early to tell yet, but I think he shows great promise.

SUNDAY 11 SEPTEMBER

THE RAIN LASHED down on the car as I started out for Glenfeshie Lodge. It being Sunday morning, as I drove through Grantown I could see the odd person here and there making their way through the driving rain to church. Sunday is like any other day for us, in fact it's often one of the busiest. There are quite a few crofters and farmers who have two jobs, running the farm and working somewhere like a distillery, so Sunday is their only chance to be there to meet us.

I used to be able to tell when it was Sunday because Jane would cook ham and eggs for breakfast. I don't even get that now. I'm not sure why it stopped, I think it may have had something to do with Jane thinking I was getting fat!

Glenfeshie Lodge is a famous sporting lodge away in the hills. Lord Dulverton owns it, but I think this week it's let to some Germans. They seem to have all the money these days; we've had quite a few staying at the various lodges around the district. They are very keen sportsmen and tend to be good shots.

Glenfeshie is an extensive estate, stretching right up to Cairn Gorm and over to Gaick. Most of it can be reached by Landrover, but they use Highland ponies to get to the inaccessible parts. When you've shot your stag, its body is humped on to the back of the pony which takes it back to the nearest vehicle, so that it can finish its journey by road. The great thing is that once the pony's relieved of its load they just give it a slap on the backside and it makes its own way home, while the ponyman hitches a ride in the Landrover. My call this morning was to one of these Highland ponies, which had gone lame.

As I drove up to the lodge, I could see Sandy Leslie's van. He's the blacksmith, and I'd arranged to meet him there because I thought I'd probably need to take the pony's shoe off to have a good look at the foot. I walked around the back of the outbuildings and discovered a group of people waiting for me. In the middle, dominating the group, was the white pony – quite a magnificent looking animal.

The ponies have to be pretty strong to carry a stag carcass over the hills, but they mustn't be too high spirited. It wouldn't be very popular if one of them ran off in a flighty moment with someone's pride and joy that they'd just paid thousands of pounds for the privilege of shooting.

I said my good mornings to the assembled group, and got the keeper to walk the pony up and down so that I could watch it. He was dressed in his Sunday best, deer-stalker hat, plus fours and all – a real gamekeeper's outfit. The others were there just to see what was going on.

I could see that the pony was pretty lame, and limping badly on its front right foot. 'How long has it been like this?' I asked.

'Two or three days, George,' the keeper replied.

I lifted the leg as he described the last outing when it had suddenly started to limp. I did what must have looked like a cross between a strange dance and a handshake, to see if it complained when I moved the leg. It didn't react at all. I took my hammer and tapped it on the foot, first the left one, then the right. When I tapped the left foot there was no reaction, but when I tapped the right it flinched and lifted its leg. At least that confirmed that it was something to do with the right leg.

There was nothing for it but to get Sandy to take the shoe off, and start exploring the hoof. It's quite a weight to lift when you put the hoof in between your legs to examine it. I hoped that the pony would help me and not put all its weight on to my back. But it had obviously decided that Sunday was its day of rest, so it leant on me solidly, like a drinker leans on a bar.

I scraped away at the hoof, looking for signs of a crack. You get these cracks in all hooved animals, and sometimes they can get infected, with a build-up of pus which causes pain, and makes the animal limp. You just scrape away up the line of the crack until you get to the end of it and the pus comes out. However, that was not to be the case with this pony. The one black crack led nowhere, so I put the hoof down, grateful for a moment's rest.

I stood back and looked at the pony again. It had given every indication of having a painful foot, but that didn't seem to be where the problem lay. I turned my attention back to the leg itself, twisting it to see if that caused pain. Sure enough, this time it reacted to its shoulder being moved.

'That's where the trouble is, boys.' I could hardly speak. The effort of holding the leg had really taken the puff out of me. 'I'll give it an injection in the shoulder, but I think it's just strained itself there. You'll need to rest it for a wee while.' I felt like *I* needed to rest for a wee while, too.

While Sandy was putting the shoe back on, I asked him if he remembered the blacksmiths Jock and Davey Terris who lived in Grantown for over fifty years. Sandy nodded and we started to swop stories about them. They were really good blacksmiths, and there are still monuments to their craftsmanship on most of the farms in the district: gates which were made fifty years ago, and still hanging as solidly as the day they were put up, not like the ones that people sell off the back of lorries nowadays.

By the nature of their job they were big strong chaps, but they were also short on temper. If Jock was in the smithy making a horseshoe you didn't go forward and speak to him; you had to wait until he'd finished, when he would speak to you. If you chose to ignore the convention, and made the first approach, you really started off on the wrong foot, and very often you'd be chased out of the door with a red-hot shoe.

Jock was quite a formidable figure what with his size and quick temper, and he also had a stutter which somehow made him even more frightening. During the war they were in a reserved occupation and consequently called up for Home Guard duties. They didn't bother to turn out because they were too busy. They

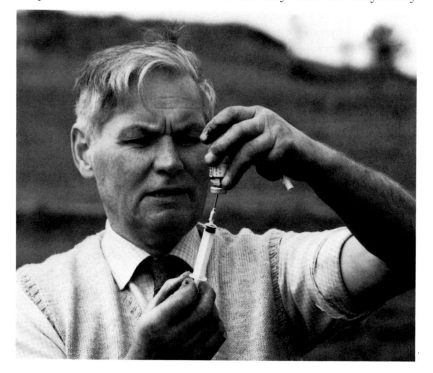

got letters ordering them to attend the parades, but they paid no attention to them. Finally they got a registered letter informing them that they had to appear before a tribunal in Elgin to explain their absences.

On the appointed day Jock went down to the court which was headed by a retired colonel with two or three other chaps on either side of him, all sitting behind a table. The colonel chap said, 'Why don't you go to the Home Guard parades, Mr Terris?'

'W-w-w-well, I'm t-t-t-too busy,' stuttered Jock in reply.

'And what are you busy doing?'

'M-m-mending the f-f-farmers' chains and p-p-ploughs.'

'And why', inquired the colonel, 'doesn't your brother go either?'

'Oh he's t-t-too busy h-h-helping me.'

'So,' said the colonel, 'you'll be making a lot of money, Mr Terris.'

'Aye,' replied Jock, quick as a flash, 'and you'll not be sitting there for damn all either!'

As far as I know they were never bothered again.

IT'S RUGGED AND windswept countryside around the lodge, and on an autumn morning like today it was quite pleasant to be cooled by the driving rain after my exertions, as we stood watching Sandy finish the job. The pony was left to rest its bad leg and we all departed.

Driving back down the valley alongside the River Feshie I saw the ruins of what used to be a small township. Strange to think that such a lot went on in this remote corner of Scotland. The Duchess of Bedford used to stay there when she came up from England in the summertime. The Duke was seldom around, but somehow or other the Duchess managed to have ten children. I know that one of her visitors was Landseer the painter, and he was certainly one of her lovers. I think he hoped to marry her, but he never did – she must have changed her mind.

Landseer couldn't have had a completely wasted time though, because he got the inspiration for his famous painting *The Monarch of the Glen* when he was there. I've driven down here before and seen stags standing up on the hill, and I must say that there's often an uncanny resemblance to the painting, almost as though the ghost has come to life and is posing in front of you.

BEING IN THE area reminded me of a client I used to have on the next estate, over at Inchrory near Tomintoul. He was mad about horses, and I was often up seeing to them. His name was Colonel Oliver Haig, and when I knew him he must have been in his seventies. He was a striking-looking man in a way, very spare in his frame and sort of gaunt. Whenever I went to Inchrory, he would come out of the house wearing jodhpurs with slippers on his feet, and the bottoms of the jodhpurs were never fastened so they used to flap about. He was quite a character, an old-style autocratic cavalry officer, who had private means. The sort of officer brought up to think more about his horses than his men.

I used to treat his horse Lucien, a thoroughbred whose sire had been a Derby winner. As you'd expect, it was very spirited and flighty, and generally difficult to handle. One time it took an infection in the hollow of the heel of its hind leg which I had to dress. It was in great pain from this which just served to exacerbate its normally lively nature. When you bent down to pick up its leg it was inclined to kick. And of course it really could kick – its reflexes were very fast.

What we usually do in cases like that is to put an instrument called a twitch on the horse. It twists the horse's nose and lip to take its mind off what you are doing, and quietens it down nicely. But the old colonel would have none of that. His was the old-fashioned attitude that he wouldn't have his horses badly used, and if that meant a man got kicked then so be it. If you worked with horses, you occasionally got kicked, he would argue; it was simply one of the acceptable risks you took for having the pleasure of working with horses.

I can tell you I didn't look upon it in that way at all. The colonel was getting on a bit and so took a while to get out of the house when he heard my car arrive. So when I went to attend to the horse the groom would get it out of the loose box sharpish; I would put a twitch on its nose and we would have finished the treatment before the old boy arrived on the scene. If I took too long I would hear the door open and this formidable, booming voice shout across the yard, 'I hope you're not using that nose twitch, young Rafferty!' Immediately I'd whip it off and reply, 'No, colonel, I'm not using it.' I don't know if he ever knew the truth, but it became a game of wits on my part at least.

For all his quirks I admired his horsemanship. He must have been quite a man in his heyday. Indeed he still was, even when he was well into his seventies. He had these fiery horses which he used to ride every day, though he wasn't fit enough to climb on to their backs, and had to be lifted on by his groom. Once he was there, however, he just became part of the horse, and no matter how spirited the beasts were, they couldn't buck him off. He was stuck there. They talk about being born in the saddle – I think he wanted to live his days there and to die there as well.

I remember one year going to call on him to see to one of his dogs. It was at the height of the grouse-shooting season. When I arrived, the front door was shut and there was a heck of a commotion coming from inside. So I went around the back where I found the keeper looking ashen. I really couldn't imagine what was going on – judging by the noise, it could have been mass murder being committed inside. I asked the keeper what on earth was happening, and he told me that it was a large party of guests, up for the shooting. The colonel had locked them inside and wouldn't let them out.

You have to remember that these people had paid a small fortune for the privilege of shooting on the estate. The colonel was too old to go shooting himself by then, but his paying guests had been out the day before and taken more birds than the colonel had thought they should have done. He'd got really annoyed about this, and when they'd arrived at the lodge the next morning for their pre-shooting drink, the autocratic old rascal had locked them in, like naughty school-children. Some of them were in a fine old rage, understandably resentful at paying through the nose for the privilege of being put under lock and key.

He kept them in until gone three o'clock in the afternoon, when it was too late to shoot, so they lost a day's sport. The keeper was none too pleased either when he saw his tips disappearing as each minute of confinement passed.

BEING THE COLONEL'S veterinary surgeon I was in a sort of privileged position and he valued my services. After I'd been on a visit one day, he said, 'How do you fancy a spot of fishing on the estate, young Rafferty?' Now the fishing on the River Avon is very good at certain times of the year. It's a beautiful stretch, with water as clear as a bell and very cold. He thought he was doing me a great honour by offering me a free day's fishing, but I told him that I didn't have the time as I was too busy. If the truth be told I don't think I'd have had the patience either.

Then he amazed me: 'Well come up and fish on a Sunday, then,' he said. It's strictly against the law in Scotland to fish for salmon on a Sunday, but this old boy didn't care a damn for legalities, and was quite happy to break the law and let someone come and fish on his part of the river if it suited him.

I was too busy on Sundays as well so I never took him up on the offer. I'm sure if I'd had the time and the inclination I could have had a fine old time.

IN THE MIDDLE Fifties I bought a new car, a Volkswagen Beetle. On my first day out with it I had a call to the colonel's place to see one of his horses. There weren't many Beetles about in those days and I'd heard stories that they were inclined to skid, so on the way up to Inchrory Lodge I booted it about a bit to see if the back end would slide. It didn't, so I thought it was all a lot of nonsense.

I finished treating the colonel's horse, and, as usually happened when he was on his own, he invited me in for a drink. I would walk in behind him, along the hallway, taking care to avoid obstacles along the way. The most difficult to circumnavigate was a huge tiger-skin rug – a hunting trophy, I suppose. It was well preserved, with the head still attached, and really quite unnerving as it watched us stepping over it.

We'd go into the huge dining room all panelled with polished wood, and sit at the end of this great long dining table. The colonel owned a chateau in France at one point, and I think he must have acquired a taste for wine because he would go off to the cellar and get a bottle of champagne ... always Pol Roger champagne. It was very good – not that I knew very much about wine then or now – and I'm grateful to him for introducing me to it, because I've been able to surprise people on the rare occasions I've been at some posh do and been asked what champagne I'd like. I've always said Pol Roger, and I think it must be expensive because they all gasp when I say it. I'm sure they must think I've got good taste for a mere country vet. If only they knew that it's the only name I know!

The ritual was that the colonel would pour us both a glass and then tell me stories of his Boer War escapades and his First World War days. The old boy's hands were getting a bit shaky and when he filled my glass some of it used to spill over the side on to this highly polished table. I was always afraid of it marking, so when he wasn't looking I would get my handkerchief out and mop it up.

I wasn't allowed to go until the bottle was empty. I think he told the same stories every time, but the alcohol somehow helped to make them more interesting the umpteenth time around. On this particular day we finished the bottle and I was dismissed. I got back into my new VW Beetle and drove off down the road. I went through Tomintoul and when I came to the bend by Craighulkie quarry just outside Tomintoul the Beetle, which had been rock solid on the trip there, skidded. And by God it didn't half skid. I struck the only strong post in the fence, which was otherwise quite rotten, and bounced back on to the road. If I'd hit it a few feet either side I'd have plunged thirty feet over the edge towards the River Avon. As it was I got away with little more than a bent bumper and hurt pride. So I vowed that if that was what champagne did to your driving I'd stick to whisky.

Colonel Haig was pretty fond of his drink, so when he bought the Inchrory estate in the Thirties, he put down a cellar of whisky, sherry and port. The whisky was kept, in the traditional way, in sherry barrels. About twenty years later the barrels were getting a bit low so he said to his keeper John Wilson that they would dreep them as the phrase is in local parlance – in other words drain them – so that they could restock them. The colonel kept the key to the cellar and wouldn't give it to anyone else, so they had to do the job together.

He sent down to the local distillery for empty bottles, which they set about filling. John Wilson said to him that they'd better label the bottles as they went along so that they didn't get mixed up. The old colonel, being incredibly stubborn, or 'thrawn' as we say in Scotland, and having set his mind on the method they would employ, said, 'Oh no, we'll sniff them afterwards and label them then.'

Sure enough, when they'd finished there was a long line of unidentified bottles which the colonel sniffed in turn saying to John, 'Whisky' (and John would mark whisky), 'Sherry' (and he'd mark sherry), and so on until all the bottles were marked.

About a week after this event I had to go to the lodge to treat one of the colonel's dogs, and as I came up the drive I could see a Rolls Royce parked in the front. As I got nearer I saw there was an elderly lady in the back seat giggling away like a schoolgirl, which I thought was a bit odd. I parked the car and, as I got out, the front door of the lodge opened and another doddery lady appeared, with her hat askew, leaning heavily on the arm of a chauffeur, who was dressed in his full livery. He had a distinctly unhappy air about him as they staggered down the steps together, in contrast to the lady who, like her companion in the car, was giggling and hiccupping uncontrollably, obviously tight as a tick.

I put the episode to the back of my mind while I treated the dog. However, on the way out of the estate I got flagged down by John Wilson. I told him what I'd seen and he said, 'Ach, the old fool got completely mixed up in the cellar the other day,' and carried on to relate the story of the bottle-filling episode. What had happened was that the whisky had been in the sherry barrels for so long that it had ended up smelling like sherry. So when these two old dears had come to tea, the colonel had offered them a large sherry which they had knocked back not realising that they were actually drinking neat whisky. Judging by the exuberance with which they left, they enjoyed the experience.

THE COLONEL SPENT half his time at the lodge and the rest of the year in Fife on an estate called Ramornie. One particular spring the colonel's caravan of cars and horse-boxes arrived, but without his wife. We were told she wasn't well and would be staying in Fife. It wasn't long after he'd arrived at Inchrory that she died, but he didn't return to Fife right away.

On the day of his wife's funeral he sent for his chauffeur Michael Aitken, and they set off for Ramornie, with Michael at the wheel. They got to the top of the Lecht which is a particularly impressive stretch of the estate, and the weather was beautiful, with the sun beating down on the river. The old colonel turned to Michael and said, 'It's too lovely a day to spend at a funeral.' So they turned around, went back to Inchrory, and spent the day outside on the estate.

As you can probably imagine, the old colonel was a very self-opinionated man. He died in 1959 and in his will he left instructions that he was to be cremated, and his ashes were to be scattered from the top of the Fairy Craggs, a tall hill on the Inchrory estate. His lawyer and the head keeper set off with the urn containing his last remains. They climbed up to the top of the Fairy Craggs and the lawyer opened the cask and started to scatter the ashes on the hillside. All of a sudden a huge gust of wind came up and blew them right back in their faces. The keeper turned to the lawyer and said with great feeling, 'Awkward to the last!'

WHEN I CAME to the district first, the head keeper at Inchrory was John Wilson. He was pretty fond of his dram. When the first grouse were shot on the Glorious Twelfth (12 August) it was usual for John Wilson to take them over to old Ewan Ormiston, who would send them by train down to London. (They didn't fly them down like they do today to rush them to the restaurants who vie to be first with grouse on their menu.) One year, 12 August arrived and after the shooting had finished John Wilson and the butcher from Tomintoul, a chap called Kelman, set off to Newtonmore where Ewan Ormiston owned a very well known sporting hotel called The Balavil. Ormiston was a great character himself; he was an Olympic shot and used to arrange shooting and stalking and so on. He was also one for the drink.

The three of them must have gone on a binge that night and drunk a hell of a lot of whisky. John Wilson got back to the estate about three or four in the morning. There was shooting the next day and no matter how he was feeling he had to turn up. The old colonel wouldn't have excused his head keeper from turning out for any reason. But the exertion of the shoot and the drink from the night before must have been too much for him. He took a heart attack and was found dying in a juniper bush.

He'd only been buried a couple of weeks when an advert appeared in the local paper for his set of new tweed plus-fours. All the estates have distinctive liveries, special tweed different from the one next door, and this was Inchrory tweed. Jock Scott, who worked on Elsie MacArthur's farm over at Ballantruan, saw the advert and went over to see Mrs Wilson. He bought the suit and was really pleased with it. He was a tall, striking figure, who'd been a policeman at one time, and he looked quite imposing in his new outfit.

One Saturday night he went into the Richmond Arms hotel in Tomintoul to get a drink, wearing his new acquisition. One of the farmers at the bar saw this disinctive tweed arrive through the door and shouted, 'By God, it's John Wilson's ghost.' He was really shaken, and it took quite a few more whiskies to calm him down.

MONDAY 19 SEPTEMBER

NEIL WENT OUT on his first solo call this morning. He's been working alongside either Willie or me for a fortnight now and we can't carry passengers, so today was his big day. His first case was pretty straightforward, a cow with mastitis (inflammation of the udder) which I saw myself yesterday. I knew the problems would come not from the animal but from Wee Dod, a diminutive straight-talking farmer who's never been one to refrain from offering his opinions, especially where the vet's treatment is concerned. Judging by Neil's report of the visit he ran true to form.

Before Neil left I gave him the same piece of advice I was given when I started on my own. If things get a bit hairy and the farmer is pressing you for an answer, but you're not sure what to do, put your stethoscope in your ears and listen to the animal's chest. It shuts out the owner and gives you time to think. I told him what I thought the treatment should be, but that he was to check it for himself.

When Neil arrived he walked across to Wee Dod and introduced himself as my new assistant. Wee Dod looked him up and down and all he said was, 'Naw, you're not, are you?'

Neil resisted the temptation to turn tail and run, and pressed on. They walked into the barn where the cow was standing, and as they arrived Wee Dod questioned him again. 'Are you a good vet, then?' There wasn't much Neil could say to that except, 'We'll have to see.'

I spoke to Wee Dod this evening about something else and he was anxious to

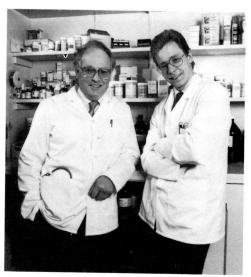

Willie and Neil poised for action in the surgery.

tell me the other side of the story. 'That boy you sent took a long time doing that cow, Raff.' It turned out that Neil had examined every inch of the animal, just to be on the safe side. Quite right too, I did the same with my first patient. You always want to check everything just in case it's not the obvious problem, and if my diagnosis had turned out to be wrong it would have been great for him to get one over on the boss. As it was he had the satisfaction of completing a day he'd been working towards for six years.

WILLIE HAD TO deal with the police today. A sergeant and a constable from Aviemore turned up with two dogs which had been caught on a farm chasing sheep. They'd got one ewe down and had frightened the others. It's usually two dogs together that do this sort of thing; I suppose it's to do with their instinct to hunt in packs.

They were beautiful dogs, a very pretty golden labrador and an Alsatian. You can't fault the dogs; it's the owners who are to blame for failing to keep them under control and giving them the opportunity to pester sheep in the first place. The effects on the sheep can be more serious than is immediately apparent. Even if the dogs don't actually get hold of one, the very action of the attack and the ensuing disturbance can lead to a flock aborting through fear. I can think of one such case not so long ago which caused a great deal of damage.

The police come to us to help gain evidence that an offence has been committed. We inject the dogs with a kind of morphine derivative which makes them violently sick. Then any signs of sheep that appear can be bagged up and used in evidence. This is all done outside, by a drain in the road, for obvious reasons!

After Willie injected them the first dog produced nothing except traces of rabbit, but the second came up with the goods – a small piece of sheep's wool, which will probably be enough to prove the case. Willie had to give a statement which will go to the relevant authorities, and we'll have to wait and see if the owner is found guilty. If he is he'll probably get a fine and either be ordered to keep his dogs under control, or we might receive a call to put them down. There is a danger that once they get the taste for attacking sheep they'll do it again, so in some ways it's best for all concerned if they are destroyed, but annoying because the dogs are not the real culprits in my opinion.

TUESDAY 18 OCTOBER

THE CAR RADIO crackled as I drove down into the valley. 'You're listening to the *Today* programme on Radio 4 where the time is five to eight and time to go over to the weather centre...'

I turned the volume down. It's hardly ever worth listening to the weather forecast; it never seems to apply to us. When I left home at seven this morning it was pouring with rain, but as so often happens up here, within an hour the skies had cleared, and were a clear, crisp, autumnal blue. A lot of southerners come up on holiday and try to ring for the local weather forecast, but there's not much point – we have our own weather system which seems to defy all attempts at prediction. It's something to do with being surrounded by the Cairngorm mountains.

With the weather so good I almost felt as though I was off on holiday. In fact I was on my way to dart some deer. There's a growing business in farmed venison at the moment, and we've got several farms in the district. Every year we have to round up the stags to saw their antlers off. If we don't they attack each other and make a heck of a mess. In fact in the wild they quite often kill one another when the rutting season starts. We have to sedate them enough to get hold of them. We can't pen them in tightly one by one as we would cattle in a cattle crush because they'd do themselves too much damage with their antlers, and I think it really upsets them to be shoved into a confined space.

With the dart gun rattling in the back of the car, I felt a bit as though I was going on a day's shooting. The main difference, of course, is that I was not aiming to kill anything, at least not on purpose! I haven't been stalking in the wild for a long time. I don't get the time any more now that we're so busy in the practice, so I suppose this is the nearest thing to it. It was great knowing that the two chaps who would be helping were good at their jobs. There's a real satisfaction in that feeling of working with people you know and trust, and, of course, like.

This deer farm is on Rothiemurchus estate which lies between Aviemore and the Cairngorms, so the scenery is fantastic. As I turned the corner I could see the stags running loose in one of the large enclosures. Alec and Jimmy were obviously a bit behind;

they'd normally have had them ready for darting in a small pen. I couldn't really go and help because my movement might have scared the animals and made them even more difficult to round up. So all I could do was sit still in the car and wait.

ALTHOUGH I HATE to be inactive for even a moment I must admit that looking across at the Cairngorms, over miles of beautiful countryside, I realised how privileged I am to be working in this part of the world. Who needs to take a holiday when you can work in these surroundings, doing work you enjoy, with people you like being with? Mind you, I don't really believe in holidays. I've only had one in forty years and that was a disaster. We took the children to the seaside and stayed in a caravan. It rained incessantly, and I don't think any of us enjoyed it. A friend did once try to persuade me to go abroad, but I can't think of anything worse. Paying out a lot of money to do nothing except get bored and eat strange food, or lie in the sun getting all sweaty, with screaming kids all around you and other sweating bodies (even if they're good-looking ones) right alongside you – no thank you. I heard something on the radio only the other day about the number of people who die just after they come back from holiday, which just proves my point! I get my holidays when I go off to inspect a zoo or travel across to one of the Western Isles to give an Agricultural Training Board lecture, or on a day like today.

The boys had the deer rounded up now on in the smaller enclosure so I drove on to meet them.

'Morning, George.' Alec, the farm manager, is a tall, rugged chap with a bushy beard, long flowing hair and deep, gruff voice. He always reminds me of Rasputin. 'They were all a bit frisky, I reckon it was that rain made them unsettled.'

'Aye, there are still two of the big stags up on the hill. They wouldn't come in when we put the food out.' Jimmy, by contrast, is shorter, neater and rounder. More what you'd expect of a gamekeeper, I suppose. His usual job is leading hunting parties off into the mountains in search of the wild deer, or showing fishermen who hire a stretch of the Spey on the estate the best place to fish from. But when there's a job to be done on the estate like there was today they all pull together.

Both men were wearing their Barbour jackets, but not for show like these townies who come up to play at being country folk. Like most people round here Alec and Jimmy have no time

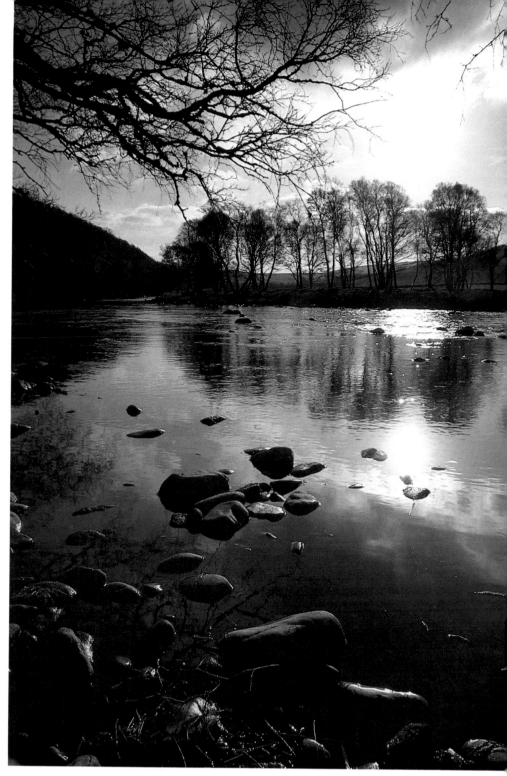

A tranquil moment beside the River Avon.

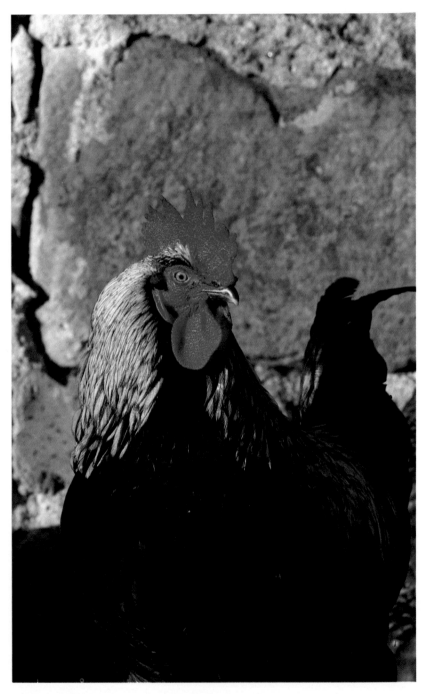

Above   *I often leave a croft with a few eggs. No salmonella in these hens!*
Right   *A familiar sight on a winter evening.*

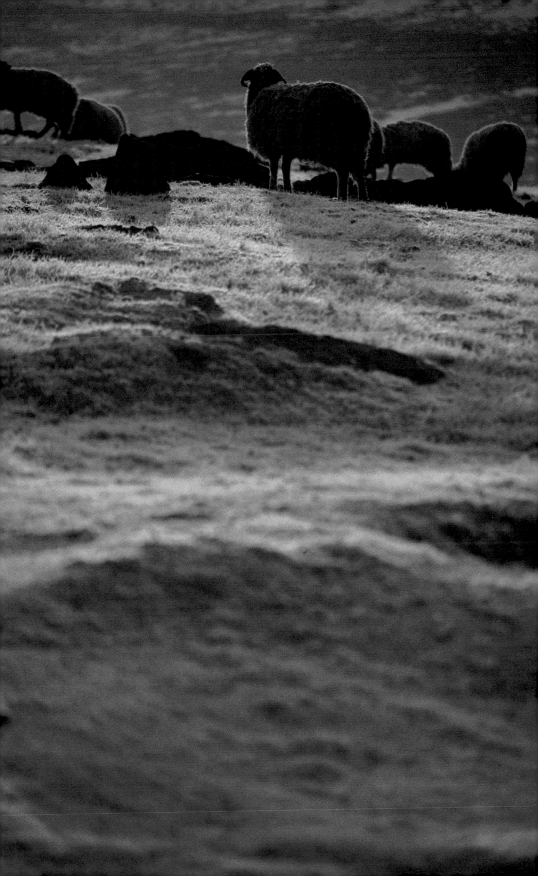

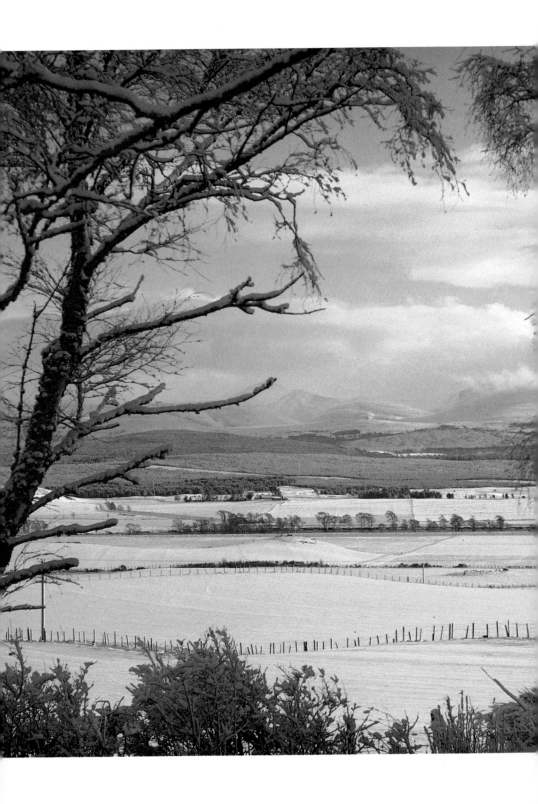

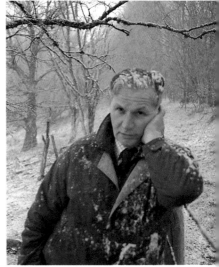

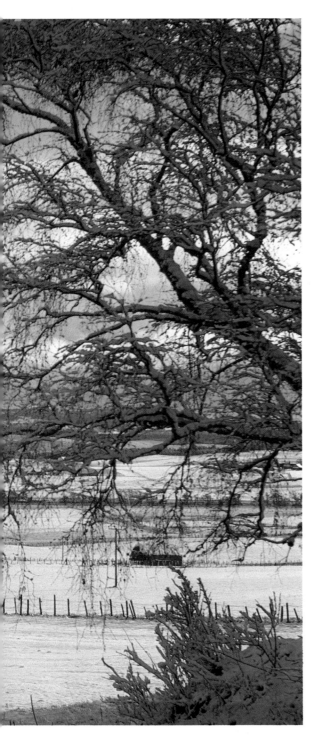

Above   *My daily walk,*
whatever the elements.

Left   *A rare glimpse*
of a snow-covered
Spey Valley during
the unusually mild
winter.

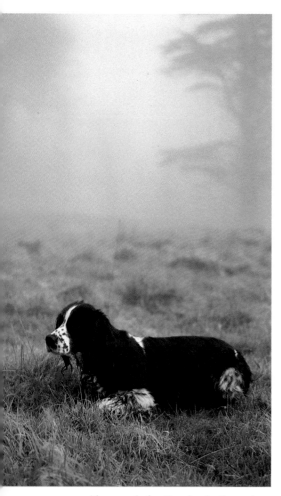

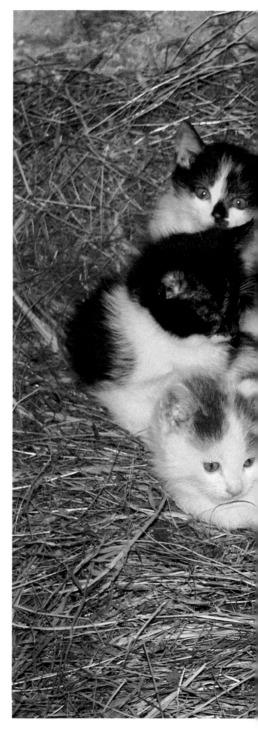

Above   *A shooting dog in the early morning mist.*

Right   *Farm kittens in Duncan Durno's byre.*

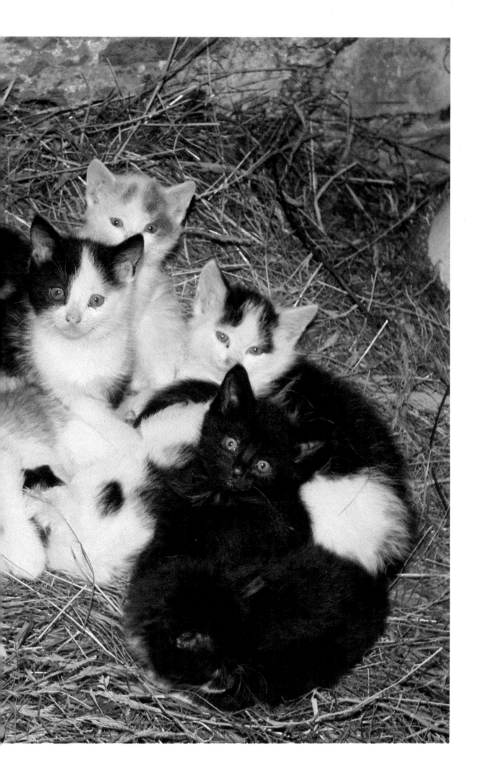

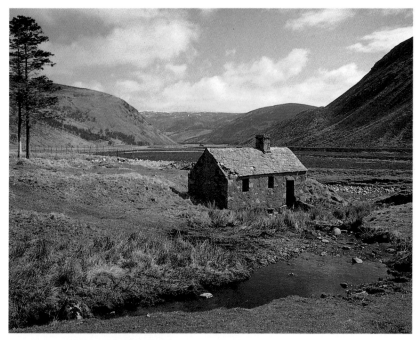

A lonely building overlooking the River Findhorn.

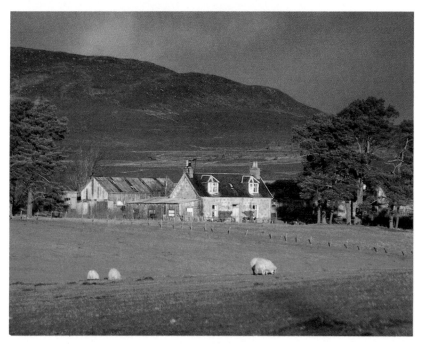

Madgie McQueen's isolated croft at Achnahannet.

for anything unless it has a practical use, and the torn and worn state of their clothes is witness to that. We've often remarked that we ought to send our old clothes down to London where we hear they could be sold for more than we paid in the first place!

'I brought my brand new saw, lads,' I said, tongue firmly in cheek, remembering last time when they complained all day that the one I'd brought was blunt. They were convinced I'd been given it by the laird to make them work harder.

'There's no need, George,' Alec replied with a straight face but a twinkle in his eye. 'We've brought our own to be sure this time!'

The drug I use to knock the stags out is called Immobilon. It's a very powerful anaesthetic which we fire in a dart from a gun. There've been several cases of vets dying after injecting themselves accidentally with the stuff. I think there was also a vet's girlfriend who used it to commit suicide after she heard that her boyfriend had been injected with the stuff. She went upstairs in the surgery and gave herself a dose of it and was later found dead. So you have to be really careful when you're using it. If even a small amount gets into a cut on your hand it can be enough to knock you out. We always carry the antidote for humans with us so that if I did inject myself accidentally one of the men can pump some into me. I hope it won't be necessary – I've never seen a gamekeeper yet who I'd like to inject me. They're hardy kind of chaps and I don't think they'd be too gentle as nurses!

With the metal box containing the darts and the Immobilon set up in the back of the Landrover we were ready to start.

'How many are there to do, Alec?' I asked.

'Should be thirty, George.'

'What sort of weight do you reckon the heaviest are?'

It's not the most accurate way of determining a dose of anaesthetic, but I needed some rough guide as to the amount of drugs to give each animal. I knew that if I gauged it correctly there'd be just enough to keep each one doped while we took the antlers off, without knocking them out cold. It usually takes only about 2.5 millilitres to put down a 3 hundredweight stag, so you can see how much damage a misfired dart could do to a human!

Sawing their antlers off doesn't cause the deer any pain. There are no nerves in the antlers so it's a bit like having your toenails cut. As long as we don't go down to the quick there's no blood and no pain. We only sedate them so that we can get hold of them and to stop them damaging us.

It's always important that my shooting hits the mark each time, not only to save me from inevitable ribbing from the others, but also because the drug is potentially lethal to anything or anyone who might come into contact with it. Each dart has a valve which opens as it enters the stag, and releases the drug under pressure into the animal. So any darts left lying around are likely to inject anything that comes into contact with them.

I think I must have been on good form this morning. The first three darts found their mark and we just had to wait for about five minutes while the drug took effect. The three of us have done this job so many times now that no instructions are necessary. The system runs itself and there is no dithering. I dart a batch of three, reload the darts while the boys work on the deer, then inject the animal with the antidote. It's called Revivon and within seconds of giving it to the stags intravenously they are up and wandering about.

They bear no ill effects afterwards, and in fact I think they feel a sense of euphoria. I've sometimes looked at one as it took a few teetering steps off to join the rest of the herd, and thought that it had a bit of a smile on its face. I'm sure they quite enjoy the dose of stimulant drug they get.

By midday the pile of antlers on the back of the Landrover was quite high. I think it's one of the keeper's perks to sell them to the local craft centres where they make gimmicky things like knife-handles for the tourist trade.

Lunch was taken in a restaurant with one of the finest views in the country – the front of the Landrover, looking out over the hills. I'm sure there's not a better place in the country to eat.

'Not a bad part of the world to live in, is it?' I asked the boys, knowing full well what their answers would be. 'There's not many bad rascals up here, and those there are soon get found out and known, not like the city where a bad rascal takes you unawares.'

'Aye, you soon get known up here,' agreed Jimmy with a knowing look, 'and you can soon take your revenge!'

'That's easy for you to say, you're a Special!' Alec returned the look.

Jimmy is a Special Constable and worth keeping in with. Before we got into any more detail I decided it was time to return to work!

FRIDAY 25 NOVEMBER

YESTERDAY AFTERNOON THE surgery door opened and a woman came in with a teenager who I took to be her daughter. I didn't recognise either of them, nor could I make out what they were carrying in a pink pillowcase, which was knotted at the top. Every now and then the improvised carrying bag twitched as whatever was secreted in it made a sudden movement.

As we went through the waiting room into the surgery she explained that they came from Aviemore, which is probably why I didn't know them. I know most people in Grantown, but Aviemore – with all the tourism – is a more transient community. As she untied the pillow case, she asked, 'Can you spay this for me, please, Mr Rafferty,' clearly not sure whether she was asking the medically impossible.

Anxious not to appear reluctant to take any work, I tried to sound confident. 'Well, I've had to treat everything from cats to elephants, so if it's possible we'll have a go.' I was intrigued as to what would be revealed when she opened up the pillowcase. From the way it was moving inside it looked as though it was quite long and wriggly. I immediately thought of my least favourite animal, the snake. People keep all sorts of things as pets these days, but the job of neutering a snake was not one I would undertake!

Before my imagination could run too wild she reached in and pulled out a long, thin, white animal. 'This is Ferrie the Ferret,' she explained with some pride. 'My husband was out in the woods and she came running after him. He brought her home, and we've had her for a couple of months now.'

I've come across this before, when someone's been using a ferret for rabbiting and lost it down a hole. It reappears later and attaches itself to the next human being who comes along.

The ferret was a milky white colour with pink eyes, I suppose it was a true albino. I got the woman to put it into one of our special white wire cages. Ferrets are notorious for giving a bit of a nip if they feel like it, so I was keeping my hands well out of the way.

Ferrie's owner left, safe in the knowledge that we were going to spay her pet and that she'd have her back the next day. If only

I'd been as confident of that myself.

I *have* operated on a ferret before, but that was quite a while ago and there were a few areas which slightly concerned me. Firstly, never having done an ovaro-hysterectomy on a ferret, I wasn't as confident of finding my way to the ovaries as I would have been with a cat, for example. Then with all these small animals the anaesthetic is always a bit of a worry. Our book containing details of anaesthetic doses and drug treatment for all the animals we've operated on would come in very handy now.

Still, I like the experience of coping with new challenges. I decided that Neil was going to be promoted to the post of anaesthetist. And ... well this seemed like a good time to delegate the job of holding the biting end to Willie.

Later in the afternoon, with Ferrie waiting in the wire cage, the three of us gathered in the kitchen for tea and a clinical case conference. A great deal of head scratching and discussion followed.

We decided to consult one of Neil's textbooks about the dose for the anaesthetic. Having a newly-graduated student around the place can be a blessing at times like this. Willie was well prepared for his task with a strong glove. We were certainly one of the most motley operating teams the veterinary profession has seen, but by the time we'd finished we were definitely one of the most clued up.

The ferret was weighed on the scales and from that we worked out what the correct dose should be. I don't like to overdose animals – you can always give them a bit more if necessary, but if you kill them, no amount of drugs will help! Neil showed great concentration in loading the syringe, while Willie tentatively put his gloved hand in and pulled the creature out. She was quite a pretty thing really when you looked at her closely. We held her between us, though I made damn sure that Willie had strong hold of the biting end, and Neil injected her. Out came the *Financial Times*, and we prepared the table while we waited for the anaesthetic to take effect.

Minutes later the ferret was limp and floppy. She reminded me then of something you'd see as the collar of a fur coat.

Now that Ferrie was out for the count I happily moved her around, and laid her on her back in preparation for removing the uterus. I was debating whether to put the incision on the side or along the belly, when I noticed something. Or rather, two things –

two enormous testicles. 'This Miss is a Mister!' I exclaimed. We were about to operate on an animal to remove the female sexual organs when it was actually male, and very much so judging by the size of the testicles.

It's quite a common thing to find that a cat brought in to be spayed turns out to be male. I suppose it must happen in about a quarter of the cases we get in. I've heard stories of vets opening up a cat and gurdling about inside for a few minutes, then looking again and finding that it's a male all the time. I can see how it

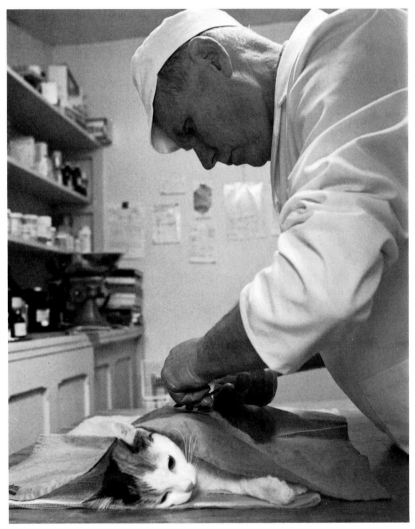

Spaying a cat.

might happen if you're in a hurry and a bit agitated for some reason, but it's one of the golden rules imprinted on all vets' brains: before starting on any operation, sex the animal. So far I haven't got one wrong, but I think this ferret was pretty close to being the first.

I'd been asked to neuter it so we went ahead and cut it, that's the veterinary slang for castration. In any case male ferrets can get aggressive when they're older so it's better to neuter them if they are going to be household pets. I can never stand at the operating table cutting an animal, especially in a situation where's there's been a bit of a mix-up, without thinking about another little mix-up to do with cutting which happened a few years ago.

I WAS BUSY doing something in the surgery one day when the doorbell rang. My son, who is a very perjink and precise Edinburgh lawyer, was staying with us and went to answer it. I heard a woman's voice and a brief conversation, although I couldn't hear what was being said. After a moment or two John came into the surgery. 'Can you cut a Cairn Terrier today?'

I ran through the other commitments for the day and even though a castration doesn't take very long, I was too busy. I told him to tell the lady to bring it back in a couple of days' time.

The following Wednesday she brought the dog in. I told her to leave it with us and come back later on. At first she asked if she couldn't stay and watch. There are times when the owner can be a real nuisance, and an operation where the animal is under a general anaesthetic is one of them, so I usually discourage them from staying. I didn't say that it was because I was afraid she might faint from the sight of the blood but simply that it was probably better for the dog if she wasn't there. She seemed surprised but took my advice and left.

We gave the dog a general anaesthetic and set to work on the castration. We removed one testicle and then had problems with the second, which was small and in the wrong place – an ectopic testicle. It was just as well that we were operating on it then, because it might have become cancerous later.

We were nearing the end of the operation when the doorbell rang, and Jane came in to say that the lady was back to collect her pet. Now I've cut so many animals, from guinea pigs to calves, that I pride myself on being a pretty quick worker, but not that quick. I must admit I was kind of annoyed that she'd come back so early and explained that her dog would need a couple of hours to recover from the anaesthetic before she could take him away. She looked slightly bemused, but agreed to return later.

We put the dog in the recovery room, and went on with other jobs. A couple of hours later the lady duly turned up. I told her that her animal was doing fine and I'd carry it out to the car for her. She said that she hadn't brought a car. I was starting to feel quite annoyed by now. How did she expect a dog which had had a general anaesthetic and an operation to walk home?

By then she was looking really confused. 'I'm sorry,' she said. 'I really didn't realise that there was so much involved in giving a dog a hair cut.'

I felt the blood draining from my face. It suddenly dawned on me that when my son had said that it needed cutting, that was exactly what he'd meant. There wasn't much I could do now except apologise and tell her about the medical condition that we'd found during the operation. She was very understanding and quite happy with the outcome and went away to get her boyfriend with his car.

When they returned, the lady stayed in the car while the chap came in to collect the patient. As he was going out the door he turned to me and said with a wry smile, 'I'm bloody sure I'm not coming to *you* for a hair cut!'

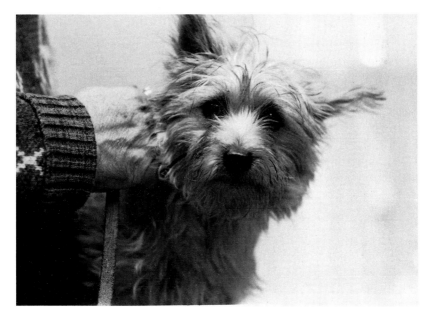

SATURDAY 26 NOVEMBER

B Y THIS MORNING, under twenty-four hours later, the ferret had made a complete recovery and had been a model patient. The only frustration was that Jane had bought it some steak, really nice looking stuff, which it refused to eat. I must try and find time later to look up and see if there have been many recorded instances of vegetarianism in the species! I was looking forward to returning it to the owners in Aviemore, which I managed to do on my way to Kingussie. When the lady opened the door her daughter was standing behind her. I couldn't help smiling as I imparted my news. 'Miss Ferrie is actually Mr Ferrie!'

Their faces dropped in amazement and the wife blushed. 'It was my husband who said that it was a female!' she blurted out. I could imagine the poor man having his leg pulled in the pub that evening, and never being allowed to forget it. However, they were pleased that we'd done the operation, and Mr Ferrie was taken away to have care and attention lavished upon him.

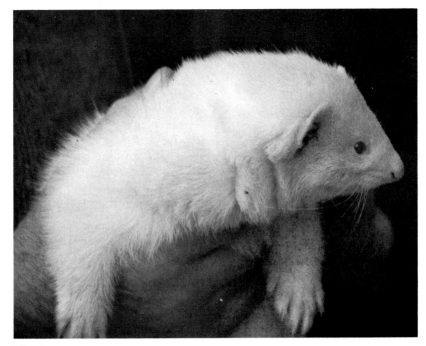

'Miss Ferrie'

SATURDAY 31 DECEMBER

As I sit in the warmth of the kitchen writing this, the work diary is open at today's date, 31 December 1988. The clock on the wall above me ticks away the fifty or so minutes left of this year. It won't be long before Jane sends me out to wait in the road for the sound of midnight, so that I can crunch my way down the gravel drive, knock the brass door knocker, and first-foot the house. In past years when I've been out on a case late on New Year's Eve, I've always rushed back to get here in time for midnight. This year I've been home for a few hours.

It's been a busy day. Many farmers try to clear up their work as much as possible, knowing that they'll have sore heads tomorrow, and I like to clear the decks of all outstanding work, so that we start the New Year with a clean, empty diary, with all the bills paid.

The year past has been very similar to the previous few years. We're very happy to have a fine new young assistant, Neil, who's fitted in very well; the work's been coming in and from a financial point of view we've done quite well. I can't help recalling my old mother saying, 'Things are going too well, something's bound to happen!' I feel that way about the practice, but I certainly hope nothing happens.

This time last year I'd have said that we'd done just about everything in the practice from treating exotic animals to capturing bears on the loose, but this year something new came along – a BBC television production team. They've been with us for a week every month since last August, and they're up at the moment filming our Hogmanay celebrations. Neil and his friends are the victims at the moment, but they'll be back with Jane and me before midnight. There are five of them and I have to say that if they hadn't been such a nice group of people we'd have thrown them out long before now. They follow us around every minute of the day and night while they're here, generally getting in the way and slowing us down. But I suppose on the whole we're enjoying the experience. We've got used to the idea that doing the simplest task such as having a meal or getting in and out of the car sometimes has to be done several times to get the different camera angles, or because we've walked too far away from the microphone. At least when they're filming us at work they know they can't stop us and ask us to deliver the calf again, or put the testicles back into a cat so that they can film it from a different position.

I'm not looking forward to seeing the end results. I'm sure Willie, Neil and particularly Jane will come across well, but I have to admit to a secret fear that some hidden aspect of my character will be revealed up on the screen. At least the programmes won't be shown for a few months.

Jane's just come into the kitchen to see what I'm up to. She can't bear the thought that I might be in the house at midnight, so she'll throw me out a few minutes early to make sure. I don't ever wear a watch – I'm always afraid that I'll leave it inside an animal I've been operating on, or inside a cow that I've been pregnancy diagnosing – so I'll have to rely on the traditional sounds which herald the New Year. We don't so much *ring* out the old and ring in the new in Grantown-on-Spey, it's more of a *shoot* out and in. At midnight the whole valley reverberates to the reports of rifles and shotguns being fired on all the farms around. So I'll pick up my bottle of whisky and wander out into the road to await the noises which will welcome 1989.

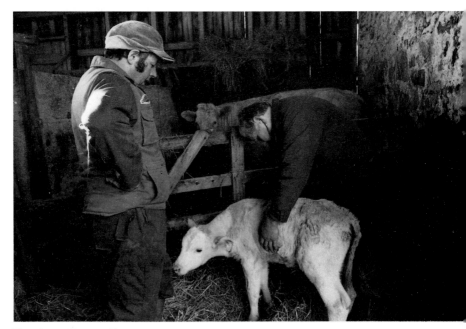

Treating a young calf.

Sunday 1 January

NEW YEAR'S DAY has been quite quiet; only a couple of callers and one call to make. Neil is off for the weekend, so Willie and I dealt with them.

Last night was a quiet night for us. I was on duty, so I didn't drink more than my one glass to welcome 1989. We have a tradition of giving presents to anyone in the house at midnight so Jane and I exchanged gifts. Jane gave me a new sleeveless pullover which she'd been knitting, and a flat cap. I gave her a new blouse. I have to be honest and say that she'd bought it for herself, but at least I'd paid for it.

A few minutes after midnight the phone went. I looked at my dram, and the piece of Black Bun I'd just started to eat, and for once I hoped that it wasn't an emergency call. I can recognise most of our clients' voices before they identify themselves, but this was a new one. It was almost inaudible, something about an emergency. He sounded a bit slurred in his speech, and there was a lot of noise which I couldn't quite make out in the background. Then the drunken voice gave way to one I recognised, Neil. He'd gone to a party at Tullyhigh, where the Hogmanay celebrations are legendary. They'd put him up to phoning, which didn't surprise me at all.

WE DID HAVE two emergency calls today, however. Mary Anne Nicolson was the first. She turned up in her father's Landrover. She had driven 20 odd miles to get to us, to save us having to go over to them. Mary Anne is a doctor down in London and with her was her friend Janet, a New Zealander who is also an MD.

'What have you got for me today?' I asked as we walked out into the drive towards the Landrover.

'It's a calf that was born either last night or early this morning, George,' said Mary Anne. 'We found it at the bottom of the field, very weak. It looks really poorly.'

Farm animals which are brought to the house are usually taken into the garage. Janet held the rear door open as I lifted the calf out of the Landrover and carried it in there. 'Pull out some of those papers, Mary Anne, will you?'

'Still using the *FT*, I see, George. It's nice to see that in this

ever-changing world some things remain constant!' Her eyes were
twinkling as she said this.

'The vet's too old to change his ways now!' I replied, not
wanting to disappoint her. Janet looked slightly bemused at the
banter. Turning to her I explained, 'I always use the *Financial
Times* around the surgery because— '

'It's the most absorbing and the most absorbent paper you
can buy!' Mary Anne laughed as she finished my oft-used phrase
for me.

We moved my first patient of 1989 on to the improvised bed
of pink. It looked strangely out of place lying on the newspapers
in the middle of the garage floor. It was a bonny young thing,
with its light grey coat and big soulful eyes staring up at us.

'Would it have survived another night out in the field,
George?' Mary Anne asked, looking intently at the creature.

'Judging by the state it's in I think you found it just in time.'

The calf was shaking violently, and you could almost see the
life draining out of it. The shock of the journey itself was probably
making it worse. I checked its temperature. It was high, 102°,
which at least meant that it was fighting the infection. It's when
the temperature goes subnormal that you have to worry.

'It's got bacteraemia,' I explained, 'where the germ has gone
right through into the blood.' I could see that the two doctors
were mentally comparing the symptoms with ones they'd expect
to find in babies. 'It's usually because they've been colostrum-
deprived, because they didn't get a suck from the mother within
the first few hours, and so they haven't got antibodies in their
system. So we give them an intravenous serum, and an intravenous antibiotic.'

'That's like gamma globulin we give to humans, is it?' I
agreed with Janet's comparison.

'But our patients are a bit tougher than yours,' I said.

'They kick as well.'

'And bite sometimes!' I agreed.

'I bet they don't complain as much, though, George,' said
Mary Anne, 'which is probably a good thing!'

I'd finished the treatment and told them to give the calf some
tablets tomorrow. Mary Anne was obviously anxious. 'Will it get
over this?'

'With devoted nursing from one MD and one budding MD,
not to mention a farmer and a farmer's wife, it should do. You

should see some improvement tonight.'

I carried the calf back to the Landrover where the engine was running to keep the heater on. It would do well to stay in there for a while in the warm before they set off again. As she shut the door Janet said, 'Mary Anne was explaining that it's worth about £200, which is quite amazing.'

'Yes, you can't afford to let it die, not that you don't want it to live in any case. It's better to have the vet's bill than have it die on you,' Mary Anne said with a twinkle in her eye.

I gave them instructions to keep it warm and give it plenty of fluid, and reassured them that now it had antibodies and antibiotics it stood a fighting chance.

IT BEING THE festive season we all traipsed into the kitchen for a quick reviver before they made their journey home. I was interested to hear that where Janet came from in New Zealand they didn't have the same sort of celebrations as we do over New Year.

'There's no first-footing or anything. We build a big bonfire on the beach.'

'One of those barbecue things?' I asked.

'Yes a barby and a few tinnies,' which Janet explained were cans of lager.

'Beer's a very antisocial drink. You're always getting up and leaving the table, aren't you?' I said. 'Whisky's much more social from that point of view, and it's much better for you as well. You being medical people will understand its medicinal qualities. Which is the only reason we keep it in the house, isn't that right, mother?'

Jane looked up from her clicking needles and smiled in agreement. I warmed to my favourite subject. 'In the old days when you had a sick calf like that, you'd fill your mouth with whisky, then go to the calf, open its mouth and blow the whisky into it.' The girls were looking incredulously at me. 'But usually the old farmers swallowed the whisky first, then blew into the animal's mouth!'

'Physician, heal thyself,' laughed Mary Anne.

'I don't think there's any harm in drink, apart from drinking and driving. I mean, we've a lot of old chaps in the practice who've drunk all their lives, and as long as you don't forget to work and eat I don't think it does you any harm. They say there's a lot more old drunkards than there are old doctors, so there might be some truth in it!' I think Janet wondered what she'd found in this remote Highland community, with its strange country vet!

We talked for a while about their work. Mary Anne is researching into cancer treatment, and developing new drugs. I feel really proud for the area that so many of our youngsters go off and end up doing worthwhile and high-flying jobs like Mary Anne.

JUST WHEN WE were finishing our drink the doorbell rang. It was John McLean with a dog which had a bad vaginal discharge. I waved cheerio to the girls and showed John into the surgery. The dog, a five-year-old plump black collie bitch, had been in before. She'd had problems with her womb, which we'd tried to cure through medication, but today's visit showed that unfortunately we'd been unsuccessful.

'Is she drinking a lot, John?'

'Yes, George, and she keeps being sick.'

I could see that she was really miserable, and knew that there was nothing else for it. I took her temperature, which was normal. That was good since it meant that we could operate with no problems.

'Leave her with us, John. I'll get Willie over, and we'll operate on her. Give me a ring about nine this evening and we'll let you know how she is.'

John stroked the dog affectionately. 'Don't worry,' I reassured him. 'We'll do our best for her.'

It's always an anxious moment for an owner leaving their animal behind. I suppose it's always at the back of their mind that they might not see their pet alive again. No one ever says that they don't have faith in my surgical abilities, but you can sometimes see it in their faces. I can understand how John felt. I must admit I wouldn't like to leave Corrie with another vet for an operation.

Willie came over and, as we prepared the dog, we chatted about the events of the previous night. Willie likes to put his kilt on whenever a suitable opportunity presents itself, and when better than Hogmanay? He'd ended up at the same party as Neil, and one of the farmers, having had a few too many, had decided to try and find out what Willie was wearing under it. He appeared to have come away from the experience unscathed and now,

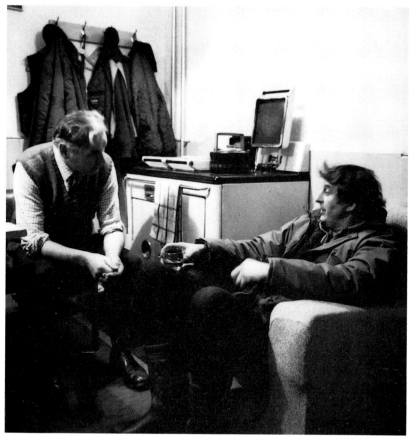

Advice and a dram with a farmer in our kitchen.

wearing his white operating coat, it was difficult to imagine the event.

The dog had been anaesthetised and was lying still on the table. 'She's young to have womb trouble, isn't she?'

Willie was right. The dog had a pyometra, which is a complaint that dogs don't normally get until their middle or old age, after they're ten or eleven. They get fluid and pussy stuff collecting in their womb, which makes them very big in their tummy. They get sick, and very often drink a lot. It's quite a serious condition because they get quite toxic with it. So we have to remove the ovaries and uterus.

I pulled the overhead light directly above the table to give us good illumination on the area of operation. The dog was breathing nicely. We tied her legs to the corners of the table to keep her steady as we worked.

Then the first incision.

'I think I've just seen what my new year's resolution should be.' Willie glanced up at me quizzically and pushed his glasses back up his nose. 'To lose weight,' I continued. As the scalpel cut deeper I couldn't believe the amount of fat being revealed. 'Not that I'd land on the surgeon's table for the same reason as this animal, but you never know when you're going to end up under the knife!'

I pulled out the blown balloon of the bladder, which Willie pressed to empty it into a tray. Then I could see the swollen shape of the uterus. It should be a pink, Y-shaped organ about the diameter of a pencil. This one was all purple and mucky, and had swollen to five or six times its normal size, so that it looked like a large German sausage. There was still a mass of fat to cut through.

'Remind me of that New Year's resolution, Willie, if you ever see me eating too much. I'd hate to think that some poor surgeon was gurdling about in fat like this inside me!' Willie smiled. 'Mind you, I'd hate to be under the surgeon's knife. If I had the choice I'd avoid them like the plague. I think we've seen too much surgery themselves, Willie!'

'Aye.' Willie had that big grin of his on his face. 'We know what goes on under the anaesthetic!'

THE DOG WAS still breathing well, just making the odd slight noise every so often. I like to hear them talking to me a bit like that. In these operations on animals which have become toxic there's always a considerable danger that they'll die under the anaesthetic. I like to keep them as lightly under as possible. It makes it more difficult to operate but they stand a better chance of surviving.

I couldn't believe the amount of fat inside the dog. 'People shouldn't let their animals get like this.'

'It's always the working dogs that keep fit and live the longest.' Willie was right. We had a sheepdog in last week for an operation to remove a growth – pretty big thing it was too. The animal was eighteen years old, and yet it was up and walking only an hour afterwards.

The uterus is shaped like a Y. We just tie off all the ends to catch the blood vessels, and then cut it out. The dog will have a sore head tomorrow, like a lot of people have had today, but it should be back to normal within a day or two.

Animals are very tough. Much more so than humans. I have to say that I was never inspired to become a doctor. They never know when a patient comes into their surgery if they are there for some time off work or whether they're really ill. When an animal's limping and lame in a leg you know for sure that there's something wrong. Our patients never tell us any lies. If for no other reason than that, I have great respect for doctors. Willie's father was a doctor, in the days when they took out your appendix on the kitchen table, and knocked you out by dripping chloroform on to a towel held over the patient's face. I can remember that happening here in Grantown. At least Willie's father knew that his patients were there for genuine reasons. He didn't have a waiting room, and they had to queue up outside in all weathers. Sounds like a good way of discouraging malingerers!

'I'm sorry I made the hole so big now, Willie.' Having cut out the uterus we were having problems getting all the fat back in, and it meant having to put plenty of stitches in. The problem with these fat dogs is that there's always a danger of the wound opening up, and they don't heal so well.

'Its respirations have changed.' Willie was leaning over the table concentrating on the dog's breathing. We'd finished at just about the right time.

'It hadn't lost much blood and it didn't have much anaesthetic so it'll stand a very good chance of survival. You go and put it on a drip in the recovery room, Willie.' As we cleaned up, the dog started to wave to us, its feet paddling in the air, a sign that it was coming out of the anaesthetic.

I HAD A look in on it again just now and, only a couple of hours after we finished the operation, it's up on its legs already. So I'll phone the owner and tell him the good news. I can't think of a more satisfying way to start the New Year.

THURSDAY 26 JANUARY

I've BEEN SITTING here in the kitchen tonight with a wee dram in one hand and a pen in the other trying to jot down a few stories for tomorrow night. Like a fool I've let myself be talked into giving the 'toast to the lassies' at a Burns Supper which the Grantown Heritage Trust is putting on at one of the hotels up the road.

Burns Night in Grantown is an excuse to have a good time. Officially it is a celebration of the birthday of our national bard, Robert Burns, and there are some who take it very seriously indeed. That's fine by me, but I'm not sure that I'll even mention Burns in my toast. I admire some of his work and though I'm not much of a reader of poetry myself, I have to admit that he was great at putting ordinary situations across in an amusing way.

There's a traditional form which all these evenings take: the haggis is piped in and formally addressed, then Burns's poem *Tam O'Shanter* is recited, followed by a toast to the lassies and a reply on their behalf. I'm sure everyone else will be sorting out quotations from Burns tonight, but I'll just content myself with a few stories about women I've known, in the true tradition of Burns.

At least I'll look the part. I phoned up the kilt-maker in Grantown and hired one from him. He had all my measurements on his files from the last time I hired a kilt about four years ago, so he'll give me the same one. I only hope that I'm still the same size – I'll have to get one of those whalebone corset things if I'm not. The kilt's the ideal thing to wear. It never goes out of fashion; it's comfortable, and you can wear it to christenings, weddings, funerals, to meet the Queen or to go to court!

In preparation for my speech, I've been trying out a few old stories on my clients. I thought I'd pop in a few observations about women. I'm sure any feminists there will throw things at me, but I don't mind as long as it provokes a response.

I love that story about Winston Churchill and Lady Astor having a real ding-dong of an argument. 'Sir,' she said, 'if you were my husband I would poison your coffee.'

'Madam,' replied Winston, 'if you were my wife, I would drink it!'

I TRIED OUT lots of stories like that on this morning's calls. No one seemed to mind them. One of the farmers said that he always liked to hear them, so I'll put them in. Then I thought I'd talk about some of the farmers' wives I've met. Most of them are really remarkable people. They turn their hands to everything, from helping to calve a cow to coping with two extra people arriving unannounced for dinner. There's a story about one of them over at Glenlivet who opened the door to a travelling salesman one day. She sat him down in the kitchen while they waited for her husband to come home from the fields, and carried on preparing the meal.

After a while two boys came in. 'These are my two sons. They're twins,' she said.

A short time later the door opened again and in came two girls. This time she explained, 'These are my two daughters. They're twins.'

The traveller sat for a minute, then asked, 'Was it always twins, Mrs Grant?'

'Oh no,' she said, still preparing the food, 'most times it was nothing at all!'

That one seemed to be acceptable as well. Then I remembered something which Jane overheard when she was in hospital having one of our children.

The minister came in on his rounds and got talking to the woman in the bed next to Jane. He asked how she was doing, and after they'd been chatting for a while she asked him if he had any family.

'Oh no, my stipend's far too small,' he replied.

The woman looked a bit taken aback, and said in a concerned tone, 'Sorry, minister, if I'd known you had a medical problem, I'd never have asked.'

SATURDAY 28 JANUARY

GOT IN too late last night, or rather, too early this morning, after the Burns Supper to contemplate writing at all. By now I've just about recovered enough to write! It was a really good do. A lot of our clients were there as well as people like Stan Hendry the local dentist. Neil took his new girlfriend along. She's the first he's had since he's been up here – well, the first I know about, anyway. She's called Maureen. I think he met her at the venison factory when she was working there over the summer. She's a ski instructor at Aviemore during the winter, so she'll be waiting for snow like the rest of them. Willie and Helen were there as well – it was a real practice outing. Willie's mum and dad manned the phones back at our house, and Neil got the job of drinking orange juice and being on call. I think it's good for the new boy to make some sacrifices for us older chaps.

The haggis was piped in by Pipe Major Ian Fraser who was telling me the other day that this is one of his busiest weeks. He's piped the haggis in at five or six different Burns suppers during the week – ending with ours, which was held three days after the Bard's official birthday. The top table all followed in behind him. I'm relieved to say that my kilt did still fit, though I'm not sure it would have been very warm on a calving case in the middle of the night.

After the meal came the speeches. I didn't get anything thrown at me, though I did notice that some of the ladies gave Jane a sort of understanding look. It was great when it was over because I could relax.

The night really got going after all the formalities were complete, and the band started to play. One of the lads playing was Davie Nicolson, whose sister Mary Anne had been in on New Year's Day with the sick calf. I was pleased to hear that it was doing well.

The whisky flowed as the night wore on. There was much dancing and stripping of many willows. Everyone let their hair down a bit, even some of the more staid members of the community. The night ended with a lift home, all 300 yards down the road, in the back of the police Landrover. The two bobbies came into the house for a drink. They were just going off duty so

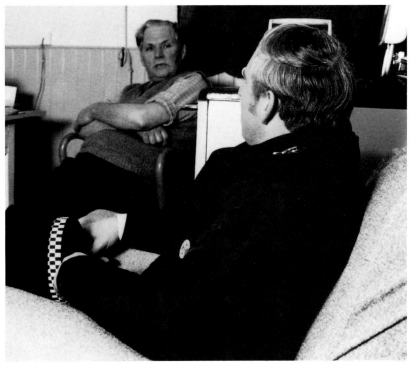

An evening visit from one of our local bobbies.

they stayed for few minutes. Jane keeps a selection of non-alcoholic lagers in the back for just such visitors. While they were there they told us that the owner of the dogs which had been worrying sheep had been fined £80 and ordered to keep the dogs under control. We went on to talk about what could be done to clamp down on it. That's the way real bobbies should work. They know what's going on around them, and they can be friendly but still keep enough distance to keep people's respect. It reminded me of old Constable Mackay again. He was a bit of a different kettle of fish, at least as far as drink was concerned.

IT'S DIFFICULT TO think of Mackay without thinking about booze at the same time. No low alcohol drinks ever passed *his* lips! He would stand in the middle of the road, this great imposing uniformed figure, 6 feet 3 inches tall, and weighing 18 stones if he weighed a pound. Invoking all the weight of the law, he'd hold up a hand, stop a car, and order it to take him to Glenfarclas where he would have a few drinks. An hour or two later he would stagger out, hold up the same hand, by now lacking some of the dignity, and commandeer his return taxi to take him home!

I remember coming back from a calving case late one night to see a group of people outside Mackay's house. I got out to see what was up and there he was having an argument with a man in a car who was obviously well over the odds with booze. Mackay, in full uniform complete with food and drink stains, told him that he had drunk too much and shouldn't drive. He knew this was so because he'd been with him the whole time and had imbibed an equal quantity.

But the chap simply told him where to go in no uncertain terms and drove off into the distance. Mackay was taken aback for a few seconds, then dismissed it with a shrug of his broad shoulders and we all went into his house for a few more drinks.

After a while Mackay disappeared into the bathroom. He was gone one heck of a long time. We shouted for him but there was no reply. Eventually we decided that we ought to break down the door to see if he was all right. We had visions of finding his huge frame slumped dead in a corner.

The door burst open and we couldn't see anything of him. I'm sure we all had a moment's panic. Then I noticed a shape in the bath – evidently in his drunken stupor, Mackay had fallen into it, and, not being able to lever himself out, had given in and fallen asleep. No matter how hard we tried we couldn't budge him either. So we found a pillow, put it under his head, and left him to sleep in the bath!

The police house was in an ideal position when he was 'feeling under the weather'. Because it was on a corner, everyone had to slow down to drive past, and just by sitting in the window Mackay could observe the cars and make mental notes of number plates, direction of travel and just about any other useful detail. If it transpired that there had been some misdemeanour committed in the area he would think back and remember that he'd seen a particular car at about the right time, going in the right direction, and make enquiries.

I suppose it's not really much of a surprise that he never rose above the rank of constable despite all his years in the force. Even though his superiors only came up from Elgin once a month with his wages, I'm sure they knew what was going on. As far as I know they never said or did anything about him, because I'm sure they also knew that he was a real policeman.

THURSDAY 16 FEBRUARY

I WOKE UP THIS morning to find that we'd had our first fall of snow for the winter. Everywhere was covered in a thin layer of powdery white. It's been so mild lately, and consequently the ground is so warm, that we knew the snow wouldn't be lying for long before it melted. Everybody's blaming the greenhouse effect for the change in weather, and certainly no one I've spoken to can remember such a mild winter as this one, not even the older folk.

It's been great for the farmers and for us. Not so good, however, for the tourist industry which is so geared up to the skiers, especially over around Aviemore. Someone was telling me that they reckon to have lost millions of pounds because of the lack of snow.

Last night's fall means that one of our perennial road hazards will be back for the next few days, skiers in cars. They'll be rushing around desperately searching for snow. Whenever I see a car coming towards me with a roof rack carrying skis, I get into my side of the road as far as I can. They drive along staring out the windows searching for any suggestion of a suitable patch of white.

The councils are so geared up to bad weather up here now that it's hardly ever a problem getting around, even when it snows heavily. The snow ploughs are out before seven o'clock in the morning, and they soon clear all the roads, even the back ones. Thirty-six years ago, when I came to the district, conditions were far worse. It was quite normal to have snow from November through to April, and the only snow plough was the local coalman's lorry. By the time he bolted the plough on to the front of his vehicle, it would be afternoon before the snow got cleared. If there was a big fall of snow there would be some places that he couldn't reach. Then the roadman would come out and clear it by hand. We all used to get stuck in and help. Travelling along some roads used to be a bit like going down the Cresta Run in a toboggan, with the snow piled up high on either side of the narrow cleared way, forming walls which towered over the car. It could be quite claustrophobic at times. There'd only be room for one car, so if you met another vehicle, one of you would have to reverse, sometimes as far as a mile.

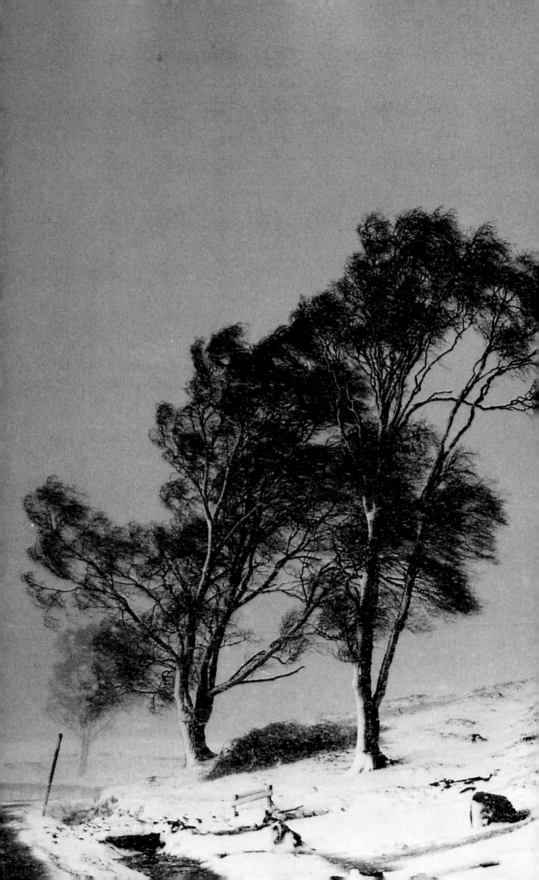

Only about 3 inches fell last night – what we'd think of in a normal winter as a pretty good day – so there were no problems. It's not only been the travelling that the warm weather's made easier. Normally at this time of year we expect to have hard frosts as well as snow, and in the past that's meant problems with drugs freezing. It got so bad one year that I had to phone the manufacturers to ask for advice. I remember phoning one pharmaceutical company about this, and the chap on the other end of the phone went away to have a discussion with some of his colleagues. He came back a few minutes later and said that it was impossible for that particular drug to freeze in the British climate. I had to tell him that unless I had gone mad, the bottle I was holding up in front of me was frozen. They never came up with any help, in fact I don't think he ever believed me, but with temperatures as low as −22°F (yes, 54 degrees of frost) it often used to happen.

Generally everything's a lot more effort when the weather's bad. It takes much longer to get around the practice. You can't get up much speed with the roads being icy, and you lose time having to leave the car in some places, and walk up side roads. The only negative side to the lack of snow from our point of view is that I'm definitely several pounds heavier this winter than I am normally because I haven't had to do any hard walking. I noticed that Willie's put on some weight as well.

The boys set off for their tasks. Neil went to the slaughter house to examine the carcasses, and Willie went to Highland Venison, where the last of this season's deer were going through. I set off for Sandy Shaw's farm.

When I arrived he was already pacing up and down waiting for me. Most people who know him call him 'Super Sandy', because he's one of the most efficient farmers around. He's built like a barn, with huge vice-like hands which can pull a beast around as if it's a child's teddy bear. He was agitated but still smiling.

'Sorry I'm a bit late, Sandy.' I apologised as I opened the car boot.

'Oh I thought you'd gone skiing with this change in the weather.' He picked up my bag and we walked into the huge modern barn. This is a farm where everything is in good condition,

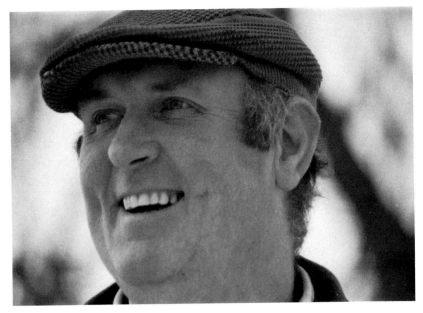

Sandy Shaw

and the cattle are well looked after. All the cows for my attention were in a pen waiting, and everything was set up including warm water.

Sandy was obviously anxious to get on. 'Right, George,' he said, rubbing his hands together, 'what I want to know is if they're in calf or if they're no; the type of bull they're in calf to; the sex of the calf; and the exact day they're going to calve, which would be a great help.' There was only a hint of irony in his voice as he said this, knowing full well that the only information the examination could give him was whether or not they were in calf.

'When did they last see a bull, Sandy?'

'The week before Christmas, about 18 December.'

'So that's the least they can be in calf – two months.' It always helps to know what size of calf I'm likely to feel. I put on my calving gown, and Sandy's big hands did up the ties at the back. I always find it amusing thinking of a great hearty chap like him doing a sort of dresser's job. Then we were ready. Sandy called the two boys into the barn and they pushed the heifers into the cattle crush one by one. I examined the first one.

'Aye, she's in calf, Sandy. About fourteen weeks,' I said.

'I thought with all your experience you'd have been able to give me the day it's going to calve, no just an approximate date, George.' Sandy was at it again. The test is a really simple one. I put my hand into the cow's rectum, reach forward and feel the uterus. If she's not in calf the uterus is a very small thing that I can get in the palm of my hand. If she is in calf, and like this one of Sandy's about fourteen weeks gone, then the two horns of the uterus are each about the size of a vegetable marrow. It's full of fluid and you can just feel a calf floating about inside the liquid. The first of Sandy's cows I examined felt lovely and healthy.

'This one's not in calf, Sandy.'

'Aye, I thought not.' He said in his gentle, matter-of-fact tone. There was no trace of cockiness in his voice, though he probably did know – he usually did. I always hope that there'll be a couple of surprises to make him feel that he's getting his money's worth out of me. He shook the aerosol can, ready to spray the animal's nose. The red marking is used to show that it will need to be put to the bull again.

The cows were nearly all through now and there were only two or three with the tell-tale red dye.

'The bull must have had a busy couple of days, Sandy.

They're all due about the same time. He must have been pretty tired when he came out.'

'Aye, George, he was almost on his knees,' Sandy replied as he opened the gate for the last one to leave.

THERE WAS ANOTHER job to do on a different cow. She was in calf and had a prolapsed cervix. In fact I could see that it was probably her rectum bothering her. The pain was making her push out the bottom passage as well.

We put her in the cattle crush. 'I'll put some stitches in,' I said, 'and leave them nice and big so that even you'll be able to see them.' A nod from Sandy.

I gave the cow a spinal anaesthetic, to keep her numb while I stitched. 'Do you think I should be shot of her once she's calved, George, or hang on to her?' asked Sandy.

I told him to see how she did. It wasn't the cervix that was causing the problem but the rectum, so she would probably be all right next year. The tail had become limp by now and I could see that the anaesthetic had taken effect – she was ready to be stitched.

I'd soon know if she wasn't. In the crates there's nowhere for the cow to lash out, but backwards … in the exact direction you're standing. I said this to Sandy to make him realise what a dangerous job we have, and how lucky he is that we don't charge danger money. He had comforting words. 'Well I think it's worse if you're standing about a yard away. They can really lash out then, but you'd hardly feel a thing where you're standing, George.' I thought to myself that if I was built like the barn door that Sandy reminded me of, I probably wouldn't. I wouldn't really like to test his theory though.

'Right, Sandy, you've seen this before. This is the ticklish bit, and I need your fingers now.' I was putting in what's known as a purse-string suture. It's like the neck of an old fashioned draw-string purse. 'Let's have a look at your fingers.' He held out his great solid hands. 'Well on any normal person I'd use four fingers, but I think I'll just use three of yours!'

Sandy put his fingers into the rectum and I tied the suture around them. It means that the rectum is held in place, but there's a big enough hole that the cow can still pass dung without any problems. 'I'll not sew it too tight, Sandy, or else you'll be spend-ing the next few weeks running round after your beast.'

'I'm glad to see that you're using nice fine thread, George.' Sandy was referring to the blue baler twine I was attempting to thread through the needle.

I wasn't going to let him get away with that. 'I know you're getting short-sighted in your old age, Sandy,' I retorted. 'I want to make sure you don't forget they're there when it comes to calving.'

Baler twine is one of the few things that's strong enough and rot-proof enough to do this job. 'I have to keep my costs down as well, you see,' I said. 'I've got to think of the bills going out to the farmer, haven't I, Sandy?'

'There's always a first time, George!' he replied.

I said that I wouldn't be able to charge him for suture material. 'No. I'll remember if it appears on the bill, George,' was his reply.

The banter continued as I finished the job. Then Sandy started to tell me about the advice he'd been giving one of the lads about working with vets. 'I explained to him that I've always found that when you phone the vet, it's most helpful if you tell him exactly what's wrong with the beast, because I've found over the years that if you don't know yourself what's wrong with that beast, there's very little likelihood of the vet finding out. But if you can tell him what's wrong, he's first class with the treatment.'

The two boys were enjoying Sandy's wisdom, which he was delivering with great weight and seriousness. I thought it was time to put the record straight. 'Well what actually happens, Sandy – and I wouldn't have told you this in normal circum-stances, but I'll tell you this morning – what actually happens is that I don't like to argue with you, you see. You tell me what's wrong with a beast, and I come and examine it and find that it's something else, not what you've diagnosed at all. But I don't like to tell you you're wrong, in case it deflates your ego. So I just agree with you but I treat it for what it's actually got. Then it gets better and everyone's happy.'

Sandy, who was listening with mock concentration, simply said, 'Oh I see,' and paused. Then he continued, 'So you're a devious sort of character as well in your own way!'

'Well you've got to be a bit of a psychologist to be a successful vet.' Sandy roared with laughter and his huge frame shook. It was infectious and we both laughed loudly. I think it would be fair to say the battle of wits was an honourable draw.

Sandy returned to the job in hand. 'Should she go outside, George?'

'Och, yes. It'll probably keep her mind off it.' I said, 'It's like these wealthy folk that get something wrong with them. They sit at home and they never get better because they're always thinking about themselves. But the likes of you and me that have to get out and about and get on with the work, soon get better.'

Sandy nodded his agreement. 'Either that or you die!'

'And if you die you don't worry either way,' I said.

Sandy let the cow out and we watched her walk away.

'You've made a good job of embroidery there, George.' I almost fell over when he said that. Until I looked at him and saw that he was still smiling.

I went inside to wash, and Sandy's wife Pat offered me coffee and Scotch pancakes which she'd just made. Sandy started on the inevitable subject. 'This snow'll no last, George. It's too warm on the ground.'

I agreed with him. 'It's been good weather for most people up to now though, hasn't it? Except I had a chap in the other night with his dog, and like I do with most people I asked him how business was. "Quiet, not much doing at all," he said. Then it dawned on me that he's the gravedigger! The warm winter's been kind to the stock and the old people as well!'

It was Pat's turn to ask for advice now. 'The cat keeps scratching her ear, George. Can you tell if she has fleas or not?' Sitting in an armchair by the Aga was just the sort of round, contented cat I like to see in a home. It makes you think that everything in the household is just fine. 'He's better looked after than me, George,' moaned Sandy, which, knowing Pat, was absolutely untrue, though mind you I think the cat does pretty well. Willie neutered him and he has a contented life now, nothing to do but sit around and eat.

I asked if he hunted. 'Och, yes,' said Pat, 'rabbits.' I explained that was probably where he got them from. 'Remind me when I go out to the car, I think I've got some drops in the boot to stop the fleas in his ears,' I said.

'Would you like a wee dram in your coffee, George.' Sandy produced a bottle and I let him pour a tiny drop in just to stave off the cold. Sandy became serious for a moment. 'I'm worried, George, that we've had all this nice weather over the winter, and lambing's only a few weeks away. I hope we don't get a bad spell then.' In the winter when it's quiet everyone accepts the snow, but when it's busy it could be terrible if it turned bad. 'We've enough to do without digging ourselves out,' he said. I agreed with him, but I don't think we'll get any real snow this winter.

As I stood up to leave I said, 'Even if the weather gets bad you'll survive though, Sandy.'

'Oh aye, we do every year. Until one year we won't.'

'And then we won't give a damn.'

THE NEXT CALL took me to Gordon Smith, another 15 or 20 miles away. The snow still lay on the hills around, which looked quite beautiful. This bit of countryside, with the Cairngorms in the distance, looks different in every season. At the moment they look like a sort of iced cake. The odd tree sticking up here and there looks like one of those decorations you can buy to put on Christmas cakes. The track up to the farm took me across a small stream, a single silver streak across the pure white of the fields.

Gordon had a cow which all three of us have been to see in the last few days. It's got a type of listeria, the same organism that's been blamed lately for causing food poisoning. Mind you, I think there's a lot of hysteria about listeria. It's an organism that's about everywhere, although it's only been diagnosed in cattle in the last few years. They get it from contaminated silage. The organism gets into the brain and causes wee abscesses, and makes them go sort of queer in the head. We don't get many cases, I suppose five or six in a year, and we're able to cure about twenty-five per cent of them if we get to them early enough. When they go really bad in the head we can't do anything about it, the abscesses get worse and press on the brain, and they just get more and more disturbed. The good news today was that this one's temperature was down a degree, and it had been eating and generally looked better. I gave her another injection into her vein, and one into the backside, half on each side. That means that she'll have a reservoir of the drug which will be released gradually to give her treatment over a longer period.

THE LAST CALL today was at Willie Grant's over at Ballantruan. When I got there I called into see another patient who I hoped would have made a complete recovery. It was the calf which was born on the day I started writing this diary. I'd had to operate on it a few weeks ago to remove the black birth lump from its shoulder. The operation had gone well, except that Willie complained that he thought I should have brought a good-looking young nurse to assist me, instead of them having to help me. It's not too long ago that these types of lumps were quite common, and once they'd been removed, the farmers used them to make ink. We don't get many these days for some reason, certainly not enough to keep even the most infrequent writer in ink.

Willie took me into the barn where there were thirty or so calves. In amongst them was the patient. She looked fine. Willie was happy, which was the main thing. 'It's real invisible mending, that, George.' I must admit I was pretty pleased to see that the wound had healed completely and that the hair was growing back over it.

Unfortunately that wasn't the real reason for going there. Willie had a premature dead calf for me to look at. It was lying in the same ramshackle barn that the first calf had been born in. Today the skylights were covered with snow, and it was very dim inside. The cow was tied up by a head chain, in the middle stall, and a few feet away lay the disfigured body of her dead calf.

Miscarriages like this have to be reported to the Ministry of Agriculture, in case it's brucellosis. The cow is kept isolated until we know one way or the other. If it has the disease, it can spread through a herd really quickly, and then on to other farms. I've had a dose of brucellosis myself, but it's pretty well eradicated in this country now. Willie told me that his brother had also had it. 'He still gets the odd flare-up, George. Sweats like an ox when he takes it.'

'The only time I sweat,' I told him, 'is when you farmers make me work too hard.'

As we looked at the calf, Willie said, 'I think the mother would have been about eight months gone, George.' He was very matter of fact about the whole thing.

I must admit that I don't like to see any dead calf. This one must have been dead inside the cow for quite a while before she aborted. The hooves were rotting and coming off, the hair was patchy. 'I thought it was where she'd been licking it, George,' said Willie.

I took the sample of blood, the vaginal swab and some milk from the cow. It was difficult to coax any milk out of her teats, but I managed to get a test tube full in the end. Throughout, the cow stood impassively,

'Will you put her away, Willie?' I asked.

'Och, I don't know. She's about four years old, so she's a young girl and she usually has a good calf. It's a real pity.'

I had all the samples I needed and gave Willie the official form which instructs him to keep her in isolation until he hears from the Ministry direct.

As I DROVE home snow was falling again and the wind was getting up. It's when it drifts that we start to get roads blocked. In past years I've arrived home only to hear the radio reporting that the road I'd just driven along was blocked. I think they put out these exaggerated reports to discourage people from travelling along the worst sections. People go out and get stuck, then the snow plough comes along and can't get by either and the whole road *really* gets blocked. So if we have to travel into a dodgy area we try and ring someone there to find out what it's really like before we set off.

Mind you, the police quite often phone *me* to see if certain roads are blocked or not. One of the policemen was telling me the other day that he'd phoned someone at the Bridge of Broon, which is one of the first and worst places to get snowed up. He'd asked what it was like at the moment and been told that, 'No one's got past, only that mad vet.'

AS I SIT here writing, the snow is falling even more heavily. I always hope that the phone won't ring on a night like this. It's quite a thought on a frosty night to get out of bed into a cold room, get your clothes on and get organised, sometimes knowing that you'd have to dig the car out of the garage before you could even set off. Back when there were fewer phones generally there was an area over towards the Braes of Glenlivet, a particularly stormy place where the only phone was in the village shop. The farmers would wake up the owner, Russell, who would then dial the number for them. As soon as I answered I'd hear him hand the instrument over to the farmer saying, 'Speak here, please.' Whenever I answered the phone in the middle of a dark, snowy, bitterly cold night and heard the words, 'Speak here, please,' come faintly from the other end of the line, I knew I was in for trouble, and more than likely a difficult few hours away from my bed.

We're not really quite in the worst of the calving at the moment, so a call tonight is unlikely, but you never know.

WEDNESDAY 22 FEBRUARY

HELLO, IS THAT MR RAFFERTY? The voice on the other end of the phone was easily recognisable as Miss Mary Kennedy. 'My friends are all all out this morning, and I was wondering if you could call in if you're passing and have a look at them.'

I told her that I was about to leave the house to go over to Aviemore, so I'd call in on the way. I knew from previous visits that early morning was the best time to see them, when they were feeding, and if I left straight away I could get there by eight thirty.

We'd had another fall of snow during the night, and most of the fields around were still white, although the roads were largely clear. I could tell that no vehicles had made their way up the track leading to the house, since it was still unmarked by tyre treads. Miss Kennedy's house is set in amongst masses of pine trees, which were still covered in snow. It was a bit like driving through Santa's winter grotto.

As I drew up to the courtyard Miss Kennedy was waiting for me. 'John's feeding them around the back at the moment,' she said in her cultured Scottish accent. She's the sort of lady who you can imagine making the British Empire great. Her demeanour is that of someone who's used to giving orders and who has spent a lifetime organising people.

She led the way to where she said we'd discover the purpose of my visit. We walked around the house along a path which revealed a magnificent view through the trees. Looking down we could see the River Spey which sparkled in the morning sunlight, and across from us the Cairngorms, covered in snow for the first time this year.

'Come on, come on. Come away, come away.' John's voice drifted around the corner of the house, and as we turned into the garden I could see twenty or so tiny creatures scampering around his feet and taking food from his hand.

Miss Kennedy's friends are red squirrels. She's been feeding them for a few years. Her interest started when, several years ago, she found a baby squirrel which had fallen out of its nest. It became a family pet, and had the benefit of the best nursing imaginable. At that time she was a physiotherapist in Inverness, which must have had something to do with the standard of health care.

I've seen photographs of her in uniform with the baby squirrel, which she used to take into the hospital. It always had a bad leg and could never have survived in the wild, but she looked after it like a child. Unfortunately it was in its run, out in the garden one night, and a weasel got in and killed it. She didn't have any more squirrels in her garden for years.

Then her gardener, John, took an interest in feeding the birds. He gained their confidence so much that all types of birds come into the garden and feed from his hand. Then suddenly the squirrels started to come back. John fed them as well and now they have a thirving colony. I'm always amazed to see John standing quietly waiting for them to come to him. He's a big chap, an ex-policeman, and I've always thought it fascinating to see this big rugged chap being so gentle and patient, waiting for the birds to fly into his hand to feed, and the squirrels which he's won over so much that they run up his legs to get food from him.

As we watched John feeding the squirrels this morning, Miss Kennedy explained her reason for calling me over. 'I wanted you to see them because I'm worried that they may not be getting a balanced diet, Mr Rafferty,' she explained as we watched a small squirrel taking something from John's hand.

I asked what she was giving them. She fished into her pocket and brought out some peanuts. 'Do you give them in their shells or shelled?' I asked.

'Oh, in their shells,' she replied. 'Their eyesight is their worst feature and I don't think they can see them otherwise.' Without any warning, Miss Kennedy turned, and rushed off across the garden, food in hand, leaving me wondering whether to follow or not. Then I saw what she was after. A small red bundle of fur was clinging halfway up a tree and she was trying to tempt it down with this tasty morsel.

Eventually it ran down, took the peanut and was gone again. Then it made a second approach and took another. Miss Kennedy stayed crouching until the squirrel had returned to its observation post in the tree, then she ran back across to me and carried on talking as though nothing had happened.

'They always like to take two. Then they run off and eat them,' she said. 'We don't feed them on anything else and I just hope that we're not damaging them in any way. You know, giving them rickets or something!' She laughed.

I had a good view of them and they all looked pretty lively. I told her that they would be quite healthy because they were able to supplement their diet with food they could pick up in the woods. Had they been in captivity I would be slightly concerned, but this lot would soon regulate themselves and change their menu if they weren't happy.

It was quite amazing to see the number of squirrels which had now got used to me and were apparently taking no notice of me, as they scampered around our feet. 'The only thing is to be sure you buy good quality nuts, because there's a disease that can be picked up from fungus in peanuts,' I warned. Miss Kennedy listened intently. 'We sometimes have problems with livestock which have been fed on groundnut meal. If there's fungus present it can affect their liver and they quite often die.'

She smiled and replied, 'These are from Bertie McFarlane's shop, and I don't think he'd want to sell me anything that wasn't first class!'

I bit into one of the peanuts, and sure enough it tasted fine. I told her to look out for any with fungus on them to be on the safe side and simply not use them. She seemed reassured, and I left to carry on with my morning's calls.

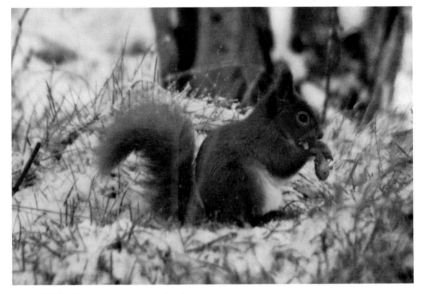

One of Miss Kennedy's red squirrels.

FRIDAY 24 FEBRUARY

THE FIRST NIGHT call during the snow came two nights later. Just before midnight, with a blizzard blowing up outside, and more snow forecast, the phone rang. I recognised the voice as that of Bertie Grant who lives on the way over to Tomintoul, on the road which can get completely blocked during the worst storms. He had a cow calving, and the calf wasn't coming out. There was no time to lose, so I set off out of Grantown where the snow wasn't too bad, knowing that there might be problems beyond the town.

There was no one else on the roads and, as always on these snowy nights, I kept wondering if the snow would start drifting further on. The great thing about night calls in these conditions is that you know you've no choice. You've got to keep going and get there because you know that someone is depending on you to come to the aid of their sick animal. I don't think there's ever been an occasion when I haven't made it, even when it's involved a struggle to complete the journey on foot.

We all carry shovels in our cars during the winter, and there've been many times when we've had to use them to dig ourselves out of drifts. I always make a point of turning the car once the spade work's been done so that it's facing towards home. Quite often in the past I'd dig it out before setting off by foot and find that by the time I'd walked to the farm, dealt with the case and returned to the car it had been buried again by drifting snow. But at least if it was already facing in the right direction it seemed easier to get yourself out. I'm sure it was as much psychological as practical.

The farmers have always been very good. If they phoned and knew it was bad near them they'd often come out to meet me in a tractor which can get through very deep snow. When even they couldn't get through, it really would be a trek, often with a large detour to avoid deep drifts of snow, taking me way out of my way across the fields. Somehow I always managed to get there, although there have been times when I've arrived and been so exhausted by the effort of the journey that all I've wanted to do is lie down beside the animal and go to sleep!

There's a story that I tell the new assistants to illustrate the depth of cold that we can get on some nights. (I'm sure some of them think I've exaggerated, until they learn for themselves by suffering through a bad winter.) It was one stormy night at about two o'clock in the morning, when a call came in to go over to Inchnacape. There was a heifer calving and the farmer couldn't manage it on his own. I leapt out of bed and got dressed as quickly as I could, not so much because of the emergency as to stop my body becoming numb through exposure to the frosty air. We don't believe in central heating, and sometimes the thermometer in the bedroom registers zero. I set off for Inchnacape which is in a pretty stormy bit of Tomintoul, with the heater on full in the car, and wishing that I'd put another layer of clothes on.

There had been a good deal of snow on the ground, but it had settled with heavy frost on top of it. It was the kind of night when you're driving along and you hear the snow crunching beneath the wheels of the car, which is good because the tyres grip, and you can fair nip along. I got to where the farm track left the main road and it was blocked by a snow drift, so I had to get out. Luckily the farmer had been watching and came down in his new tractor to pick me up. I remember being amazed at how cosy the inside of the cab was. It was one of the latest models with a fan heater blowing from the roof and a radio playing – a limousine of tractors.

I'd have stayed in there out of choice, but there was a patient to be seen. The farmer took me into the byre and I examined the cow which was standing there with great clouds of steam forming at her mouth every time she breathed. The calf was too big to calve in the ordinary way, so I knew that it would have to be a caesarian section.

I sent the farmer into the farmhouse to get his wife, who came out to help, which was a great bonus because she was a district nurse and had an idea of what to expect at least. She brought the bucket of warm water for us to wash in, and I put the instruments into hot disinfectant in a basin. We'd only been working for a few minutes when I noticed that a crust of ice had formed on top of the water in the basin, which shows how cold it must have been. I had to break through it to get the instruments out, but it didn't seem to cause too many problems and we got the calf out alive.

When it came to stitching up the heifer we encountered a new, unforeseen problem. Every time she breathed, air was being forced in and out of her abdomen. As soon as this hit the cold night air, the water vapour in it formed into a mist which got worse with every breath. In the end I had an awful job seeing the wound; it was like operating through a dense fog!

I managed to get the wound stitched up, but it took some time. I'd been moving around quite a bit, and hadn't noticed how cold it was, until I finished and looked at the farmer and his wife who'd been standing still holding the animal and the wound. Their faces were deathly white, as were their bare hands, which had lost all sign of blood. Then the cold hit me too, and I started shivering and shaking uncontrollably, and some of the drops of sweat which had formed on my face froze.

We couldn't take refuge in the warm kitchen until we could see the cow had started to lick the calf. It's such a strong part of their maternal instincts that they usually do, But it's even more important in that degree of cold. The rough tongue not only cleans the calf, but also dries it. If that doesn't happen the calf is left with moisture on its coat, which, in very cold weather can lead to frostbite. We often see calves with the tops of their ears missing because of frostbite. It certainly spoils their looks, but there's not a lot we can do about it. If their legs are left wet then eventually the hooves can drop off which is obviously a lot worse. This mother was doing her bit, so we beat a hasty retreat into the farm kitchen for a mug of tea and a dose of the best traditional medicine, a dram of The Glenlivet, specifically designed to cope with just these sorts of emergencies.

I found it a bit hard to face leaving the warmth to make my

way back, but it wasn't too bad because the farmer took me down to the car by tractor, and I suppose I got back to the house at about eight o'clock just in time to take the first of the morning's calls and start a new day's work. Jane had a good hot breakfast ready for me, which helped to keep my spirits up for the rest of the day.

I was discussing night calls with one of the local doctors, and he said that he just pulled his clothes on over the top of his pyjamas, so that when he returned from the call he didn't have to put on cold pyjamas, but could just peel off the outer clothes and leap into bed. Better for self and partner. I thought this made a lot of sense, and had every hope that it would solve all that was worst about night call-outs. So the next time I was dragged out in the small hours to a calving case I did exactly as the doctor had suggested.

It was a cold, frosty night, and I got to the farm where I found the cow in dire need of my attention. Off came my jacket, and I started to roll up my sleeves. At which point I discovered something infuriating about pyjamas, or at least the ones Jane buys for me. The sleeves are made so tight that it's impossible to roll them up.

This would not be the sort of problem which would keep most men lying awake, but for me at that moment things were different. Within a few seconds I was going to have to shove my arm deep into the cow, so any lengthy ponderings were out of the question. There was nothing else for it but to strip right off, removing shirt and pyjama top, then get back into the shirt, roll the sleeves up and start to calve the cow. So instead of keeping the pyjamas and me warm, ready to leap back into bed on my return, I lost more heat than I would ever have done if I'd stuck to my usual dress.

That doctor's ears should have been as red as my chest was blue that night, with the amount of curses that I directed at him and his wretched ideas. I suppose I should have thought that doctors don't often have to roll up their sleeves to examine or treat their patients, even when they are giving birth.

I DIDN'T WEAR my pyjamas last night, but I was well prepared for the dirty weather. The wind drove the snow horizontally into the windscreen, and made it drift across the road in places. The further I travelled the worse it became.

About half a mile away from the farm I started to get stuck.

Every few hundred yards the car would veer off violently as the wheels lost their grip. It's a heck of a job to keep it on the road, wrestling with the wheel to counteract the skids. You have to keep up a steady speed – not too fast though – so that you use the car's momentum to push through the small drifts. I got stuck at one point in the ruts made earlier in the day by a tractor. It's one of the hazards which often foil us. The ruts are so deep that the bottom of the car rests on the snow and the wheels can't grip. All that you can do is get out and dig away as much of the snow from underneath the chassis as possible so that the weight of the car helps to gain traction.

I switched the torch on and looked underneath. The car was well and truly stuck, but I could see that as long as I could get out of this drift, the road immediately ahead would be passable. When the snow is powdery it's easy to drive through in the first place, and also easier to shift when you have to. Unfortunately this was compacted wet snow, which is heavier to shovel away.

After clearing the snow I got back in the car and used the clutch to rock it to and fro, eventually managing to get enough momentum up to get over the top of the rut.

Back on the road there was no great problem until I got about half a mile away from the farm. I could see the lights in the distance through the blizzard, but I knew that the car was not going any further. I tried to drive through a huge drift across the road, but it just got well and truly stuck. The only thing to do was to reverse out of it, park the car as far off the road as possible and walk.

I set off with my Gladstone bag containing my calving gown and, I hoped, all the instruments I'd need. It was one of those walks you see people do in old silent movies, leant forward at forty-five degrees, just to stop being blown over. I had to walk right into the teeth of the blizzard, but at least I could console myself with the thought that to get back I'd have a large hand pushing me.

Bertie was in the byre when I arrived. His hair was tousled, looking like the straw on the floor of the barn. 'Sorry to get you out on a night like this, George,' he said as he pushed his hand through his hair and rubbed his eyes. He looked as though he'd not been awake for long.

I never cease to be amazed at the stamina of some of these farmers. They take a lot of care to ensure that a calf is born alive

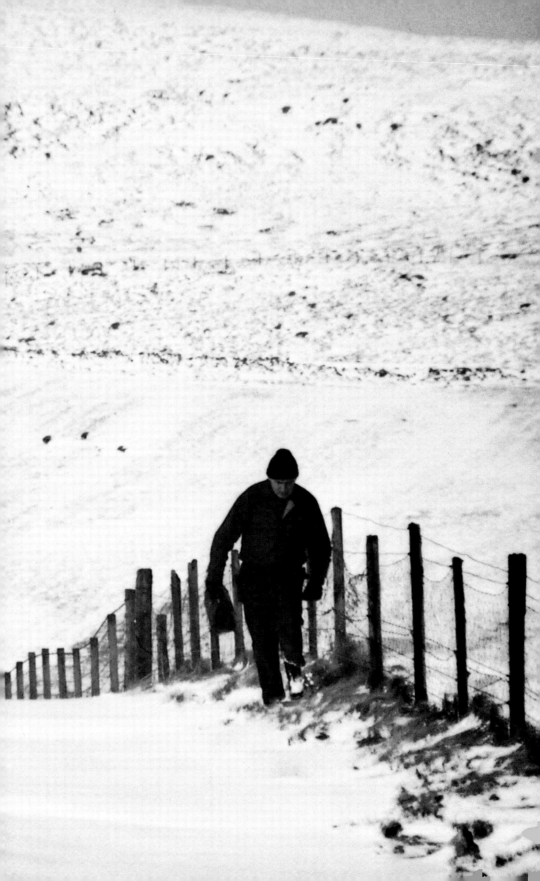

and it's not at all uncommon to find them getting up two or three times during a night to look at their cows during the calving season, in order to check if any of them are needing help. Some of these farmers who are on their own can do that for weeks on end when they have a large herd to watch. They get up, have a wander round, and then go back to sleep again.

BY THE LIGHT of the single overhead bulb, I could see that Bertie's cow was pressing hard, and that there was no time to lose. A quick examination inside her told me that the calf's head was twisted, which was why it wouldn't come out. Without too much difficulty I managed to manipulate it enough to pull the two forelegs out a few inches, enough to tie a rope to each leg. 'Right, Bertie, you take this one,' I said, handing him one of the ropes, 'and pull.'

We both put our backs into pulling, but it was obvious that the calf still wasn't going to come out. 'I'll have to use the eyehooks, Bertie.' I rushed to my bag and pulled out two more smaller ropes with the hooks attached. These go into the corner of each of the calf's eyes. When you pull on them it has the effect of pulling the head down on to the legs so that they are in line. You then pull on the other ropes at the same time and the calf slips out, a bit like the way you see Superman flying on all those comic strips. It sounds horrendous, but the hooks are not like fishing hooks – they're very large and rounded. Their smooth surfaces pull on the bone of the eye sockets just enough to keep the head down, and do no injury whatsoever to the calf.

We both pulled again and after a few anxious moments when I thought it really was going to get stuck, it started to slip out. From then on it came out smoothly with hardly any trouble at all. Five minutes later it was on the hay being licked clean by the mother, and we went inside to get washed and for a small something to build up my reserves for the walk back to the car. It was only about half past two, so I knew I'd be back before dawn, ready to start another day's work.

FRIDAY 3 MARCH

TWO OF MY calls today brought home to me how varied our work up here is. They were jobs which have more of an environmental health role than a veterinary one, although in Scotland the two are more closely linked than in England and Wales. One call was to the Highland Venison factory, the other to the smoked salmon factory in Cromdale, a village just outside Grantown. The girls who do all the filleting and packing of the salmon are usually good for a laugh, and it's not too arduous a job, so it was just what I needed.

Our duties at the factory involve checking throughout the year for general hygiene standards, and certifying the quality of any smoked salmon which is being exported. The company used to be owned by one of the local distilleries, but it's just been bought by a chap called Ian Anderson who I gather is a rock star in a group which delights in the name of Jethro Tull. I met him the other day for the first time and he wasn't anything like I expected him to be. I thought that being a rock star he would be sort of way out and weird, but he's a real businessman, and he's obviously taken a lot of time and effort to get to know exactly what's going on in this particular type of business. He was telling me that he's got similar ventures in other parts of Scotland, and I was really impressed; he seemed to know what he was talking about as far as the factory and his plans for it were concerned.

Today the factory had an order going off to America, which I had a look at. It's great to think that someone in a top-class restaurant across the Atlantic will be sitting down soon to enjoy the delights of the Spey!

To see the girls at work is quite amazing. There's one, Dolly Gordon, who was sent to Japan last year to show them how to fillet and slice fish, which was quite an honour and a real case of coals to Newcastle. I always feel sorry for the one boy in there. He must have a hell of a time – all those girls to tease him all day.

From our point of view it's not one of the most financially rewarding elements of the practice, but it gives me a lot of satisfaction to realise that we're helping to keep one of the local employers going. If it were to close the effect would be more damaging in the long run than just the twenty or so jobs which would disappear. It's the only employer of women in Cromdale, and therefore an important way of keeping women in the area. In some areas where there aren't jobs for women, the young girls leave to look for employment. Then it's not long before the young men follow.

I've seen this happen out on the Western Isles. There are communities with just middle-aged single men, because the women have left in search of jobs. Eventually the community will die because there are no youngsters coming along to keep the cycle going, and to support the old folk. So any woman searching for a good-looking man need only take the short ferry-ride across to Lewis where they'll find plenty of eligible bachelors to choose from.

ANOTHER OF THE routine jobs we have is at the Highland Venison factory. They take in carcasses from all over the area, deer that have roamed the heather hills, and strip and prepare them ready for the butchers. We examine each carcass and give them a certificate for export. Willie had been hard at work there since early morning – it's a busy time at the moment.

I have what I suppose is a bit of a bee in my bonnet about venison from the health point of view. It's one of the most healthy meats you can eat, low in fat, because the fat is not marbled throughout like it is in beef, but on the outside of the cuts and therefore easy to trim off. I've persuaded them to make health sausages, using no animal fat, but Flora margarine. This means that they are high in polyunsaturated fatty accids and a lot kinder to the arteries. As I left, Kerry, the manager, proudly thrust half a pound of them into my hand, so that I could consumer test them.

AT HOME IN the kitchen I presented Jane with the sausages. The boys were there writing up their day's notes. 'How did you get on with the navel, Neil?' I asked. I'd sent him off to investigate a vague message we'd received about a calf with something hanging down from its navel.

'When I got there I thought it looked like a bit of baler twine from a distance. I thought I might have discovered a new medical condition,' explained Neil with a smile. 'But as soon as I got closer I could see that it was just an infection, and it was the mucus dangling down.'

Willie had been to test some Highland cattle at the

Rothiemurchus estate. 'They were really frisky,' he said. 'I think they get excited by the white everywhere.'

Then Neil gave a big grin, looked very pleased with himself, and announced, 'Tomorrow it'll be six months to the day since I arrived.' It just shows how quickly the year's going. I called Jane in and we had a drink to celebrate. Neil's now doing really well. I think he's learnt a lot from us two old hands, and we've learnt a few things from him as well. He's turned out to be every bit as good as I'd hoped he would be. I think he's getting keen on his girlfriend, so who knows what might happen.

I REMEMBER A girl I courted when I was in my first job. It was in Suffolk just after the war. I went to work for a chap called Geoffrey Muir who was quite a formidable vet. He'd gone to Canada to seek his fortune and qualified as a veterinary surgeon there. When the First World War started he came back to England and was commissioned. He won the Military Medal in one of the campaigns, so I really looked up to him.

When I was appointed he said that he'd arranged digs for me, which I thought at the time was very kind. They were about three or four miles away from the practice, so pretty handy. The only drawback, and quite a considerable one as it turned out, was that they were with the local vicar. Although I'm not a religious person, the fact that he was a man of the cloth was not the problem. It was the man's character and the rather impecunious circumstances he was in which caused me problems.

When I turned up at the rambling vicarage, I expected a warm, smiling, possibly slightly batty vicar who would offer me a sherry and engage me in gentle theological debate. I was not prepared for the Reverend Martin Black, a small man who was more than a little odd, and very self-opinionated. For some strange reason which I never discovered he was also a fellow of the Royal Geographical Society.

As he showed me around the vicarage I couldn't help noticing a distinct lack of furniture and fittings. Being a young graduate, however, I didn't feel it was my place to inquire as to the reason for the lack of home comforts. In fact it was only after several days spent there being fed on baked potatoes by his wife, who was very nice, that I discovered the reason for his state of poverty. One of the farmers who I called on filled me in on the details while we were standing in a barn castrating calves. As the story unfolded

I took increasingly less interest in what I was doing and more in the tale, to the extent that I cut my hand.

In those days vicars received nearly all their income from the wealthy members of their flock, mostly local landowners, but Reverend Black's monthly receipts were on the small side to say the least. He'd fallen out with most of his parishioners a few years before and had to take in veterinary assistants to make ends meet.

I had to wait a few days to prise the rest of the information out of another farmer, and this time I was more careful to stop what I was doing while he completed the picture. The Reverend gentleman had never been a favourite in the area. He was too fond of his own views, and the congregation had already been dwindling, when a series of events occurred which turned the whole neighbourhood against him.

One of the local girls wanted to get married but decided she didn't like the Reverend Black, so she went to the neighbouring parish instead. The Reverend was pretty furious about this. A year or so later the couple had a child, which they had baptised in the same neighbouring church. Unfortunately the child died and the woman decided that she wanted it buried in her own parish, but the Reverend Black was not going to show any compassion. He said that it was just retribution for her not having married and had her child baptised in her own parish, and wouldn't allow the burial in his churchyard. The girl decided to contest this, in an attempt to win the right to bury her child in her home town. The case went through all the ecclesiastical courts and the Reverend had to finance lawyers to defend himself and fight the case. The only way he could do this was to sell everything in his house to raise money – there was certainly no one in the area who would have helped him.

He lost the case and the child was laid to rest in his churchyard. But when the mother wanted to erect a memorial stone, it transpired that the Reverend had the power of veto over what form the memorial could take, and he wouldn't approve any of the ideas put forward. The family took him to court again, but this time they lost the case, so nothing was ever erected.

Understandably this created bad feeling in the district and he lost virtually all his congregation, which had already been on the light side, and therefore also his income. He dragged me along to a service one Sunday and more noise came from the woodworm in the pews than the worshippers. I think there were just three other people in the church: an old lady who was deaf, and two people on holiday. None of which would have helped his income.

He had a son and two daughters, one of whom I ended up walking out with a few times. I think I felt a bit sorry for her, having this strange vicar for a father, but she took after her mother and was very pleasant, so it wasn't too much of a chore. None of the locals were very keen about venturing up to the vicarage even to see the daughter, so I think I was a bit of novelty. Suddenly I realised that I had become more than that in the vicar's mind and that he saw in me a future son-in-law and possibly the answer to his financial problems. I definitely wasn't interested in hearing wedding bells, not that they could have found enough people in the parish willing to ring them, so I thought I'd better get the hell out of it before it all got too involved.

I moved into new digs, hoping that the move would avert any danger of being married off. However, I wasn't to get away from his attempts at matchmaking so easily. This old character used to ride down to my lodgings on his bicycle, cassock billowing and straw hat perched precariously on his head, kept from flying off by an old piece of string tied firmly underneath his chin. He would arrive at the house at all times of the day and night, knock on the door and demand to see me. My landlady, who was a good old sort, always used to say that I was out, and he'd cycle off again. Then she'd come in and say, 'That bloody vicar has just been in again.' Thankfully he got fed up with pursuing me before my landlady tired of protecting my bachelorhood, and I got off that particular hook. I never saw the daughter again anyway.

I'm sure Neil won't have the same problems as I did, that's one thing.

TUESDAY 7 MARCH

I WENT TO Laggan today to treat some cattle, and a chap called Winston was there helping. We got talking about his old boss who was called Alex Herbage. He was quite a character who turned out to be substantially different from the image he projected.

When he arrived on the scene about ten years ago, Donald McKinley, the estate manager, phoned me up to say that the Dalchully estate had been bought by this chap Herbage. I asked him what he was like, and Donald said, 'Very fat!'

'Does he have a wife?' I said.

'Aye,' replied Donald.

'And what's she like,' I asked.

'Very flat!'

When I met Herbage for the first time I could see what Donald meant. He was a big man in every sense: his lifestyle was flamboyant, his aspirations were great and his size was enormous. His last recorded weight was 35 stones!

As far as we knew he had made his money from financial ventures, including offshore investment companies which he set up in exotic places like the Cayman Islands and the Bahamas.

I first met him when I was called across to look at some cattle. I don't think I've ever seen such a fat man. He was quite odd to look at – he had a tiny head for the size of his body, his huge arms wobbled as he moved, and yet his wrists and hands were normal size with tight skin, almost as though he'd put a strong elastic band around his wrist to keep the fat up his sleeves out of the way. He was quite a charming man to meet and although as it turned out it was all a con, he was quite a likeable character.

We met him socially when we were invited to a Highland Games that he ran one year. I remember him arriving escorted by bagpipers, just like the laird he so desperately wanted to be. It was quite a grand affair, I think most people went along to see the 'Fat Man' as he was generally called. Jane and I were invited to the official lunch party at the house.

It was one of those fancy lunches with cocktails and tiny bits of food on trays. I don't know how he managed to satisfy what must have been a huge appetite, but I like to have a good lunch and I was still hungry at the end of it. As soon as we could get out we wandered off in search of more food.

Out in the field there were all sorts of food stands, and a lovely smell was coming from a stall selling venison burgers. There was a long queue so I wandered off round the back and met Donald, the estate manager. I told him that I was after a burger, and asked him where they'd bought them from. 'Oh they weren't bought,' he said with a rueful smile. 'I had to make all two thousand of them myself!' He went on: 'I started to make them in a basin, but I wasn't getting anywhere so I used our bath instead.'

My hunger left me all of a sudden. 'I'm glad I didn't get to the front of the queue in that case, Donald,' I said. 'I'm not sure I fancy the idea of food made in your bath!'

He laughed. 'Oh it was worse than that,' he said. 'Just when I'd got all the ingredients mixed together the wee toddler came along and fell in amongst it!'

That really put me off, and I stayed hungry for the rest of the day – unlike Alex Herbage who was there in the afternoon watching the games. When he got hungry, he sent Donald off for some of these 4 ounce burgers. Nobody could quite believe it, as he sat there and ate fifteen of these substantial offerings.

It must have been in 1984 that his world fell apart. All of a sudden there were stories in all the papers about the 'Fat Man'. The bubble had burst on all his financial deals and he ended up in Pentonville Prison awaiting extradition to America, where he faced charges of defrauding American investors out of 46 million dollars. That was only the tip of the iceberg, it turned out that he owed over $200 000 000 in total. But the charges were enough to get him a possible 135 years in jail and fines of $43 000, so I suppose they didn't bother with the rest. It turned out that his whole life had been a succession of cons and that he'd been convicted on several fraud charges earlier in his career. His main way of making money was to take investments from people, and siphon off the bulk of the cash into his own accounts, then use money from new investors coming into the schemes to pay off the existing ones when they wanted to get out. I can't imagine how he thought that he'd ever get away with it. I'm sure the answer must be that he began to believe everything he said, to such an extent that he no longer saw it all as a fraud. The last thing I heard he was in a jail in Florida serving his sentence.

FRIDAY 17 MARCH

TODAY TURNED OUT to be one of those frustrating days. It started innocuously enough with a trip up to Tomintoul to do some routine cattle testing – a job I don't mind doing even though I must have done thousands upon thousands over the years. If the company is good and there's plenty of good crack, it can be great fun. I was trying to explain the meaning of 'crack' to an Englishman the other day. It's one of those words in Scottish dialect for which it's difficult to think of a direct translation. I suppose it means gossip, but that somehow sounds inadequate.

Hamish McIntosh, who runs a small farm, arranged for some of his cattle to be castrated and others to be tested for tuberculosis. This is one of the Ministry of Agriculture required tests, and usually a mere formality. We haven't had any TB for years up here, but the tests still need to be done.

It was a bit of a social event and two of Hamish's neighbours, Willem Sheed and Willie Turner, were there to help. We were in the local market, using the cattle crush. It's a very simple affair. just a narrow corridor of fencing down which the beasts go. They're stopped at one end by a gate and then another gate is closed behind them. We put a halter on them, which is tied to the framework of the crush. The animal is held in a confined space, unable to move about too much, so it's easier to work on than if it were just tethered by the head and free to thrash around. In this small community the local market is only used for sales on a few occasions a year; the rest of the time the farmers use it for work like this. It's real team work: one of the men operated the gate and put the halter on, the second drove the cattle in and shut the back gate, while the third kept the record of what we did.

The test is a very simple one. We inject tuberculin in two places and go back three days later to see if there's been any reaction to either injection. We know by the reaction whether the animal is infected. The cattle have numbered ear tags which are supposed to be unique, and identify the beast from birth to death.

I noticed Hamish was wearing one of those bleeper things, looking incongruous on his belt alongside some baler twine and the rope for a halter.

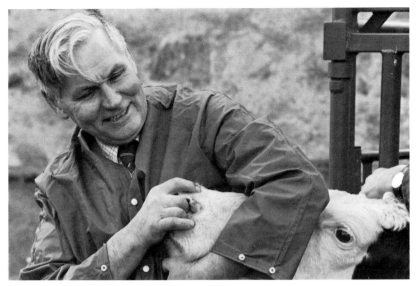

Getting to grips with a patient.

'You becoming one of those yuppies, Hamish?' I must admit I like to try and get people going sometimes just for the sake of it. And there's nothing like suggesting they're becoming gentrified to annoy someone like Hamish!

'Ach!' came the concise reply.

'Get on with you, George.' The others were warming to the idea. 'It's one of those electronic tags like they want to use for prisoners, for the wife to keep track of him.'

'You'll be the one laughing if it goes off, George!' I could see that Hamish knew he held the punch line. 'It's my Fire Service bleeper!'

Willie joined in. 'You'll be here on your own if that happens!' He pointed to his own gadget tucked firmly underneath his water-proofs. I knew that the three of them were part-time firemen for Tomintoul; they'd never been called out yet when we'd been working together, but there's always a first time.

'Even if you were in the middle of a castration with one testicle half out, we'd be gone, George,' were Hamish's comforting words.

LUCKILY THERE WEREN'T any fires in Tomintoul today, so we managed to get through all the work very quickly, and I was able to get home early for lunch. When I arrived Jane was with

Mark, one of our six grandchildren. Anne, our second daughter, married a local farmer, John, and they live nearby in Nethybridge. At the moment Anne is doing a business course in bookkeeping for three days a month. Sadly, Mark has a form of cerebral palsy which means that he takes more looking after than a four-year-old usually would, so Jane has him to stay overnight once a week. He's a beautiful child with masses of curly blond hair, and he's always a hit with everyone who comes in.

Jane broke some news to me that she knew would put me in a bad mood. 'Davie Nicolson phoned to say that they've got a cow bulling.'

This may not sound like the sort of information which could make anyone tetchy, but I knew what lay behind the information. I ate the soup Jane put in front of me, hardly trusting myself to say anything. I could feel the tension growing inside me.

Davie had bought a bull from a stock sale nearly three months ago and it hadn't been performing up to scratch. It had been bought with a guarantee which means that if there are problems within twelve weeks of the sale – and the buyers can provide evidence of them – they can get their money back. This particular bull had been serving cows with no problem, but hadn't left any pregnant.

I'd known that the call was likely to happen at any time because the guarantee period was nearly up. In the summer, cows

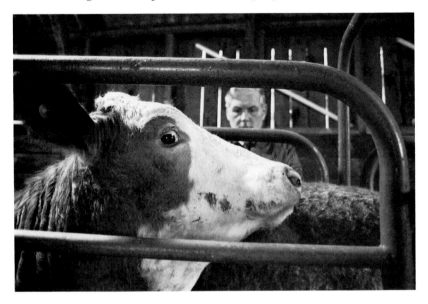

stay on heat for up to twenty-four hours, but in the winter it can be as little as a couple of hours, so when the call comes there's no hanging about. I wolfed down my lunch with hardly another word. Jane knows me well enough not to take any notice of my mounting tension.

DRIVING TO THE farm I thought of other occasions when I'd performed this particular duty, which (in my defence) some vets refuse to undertake. The job is to get a sample of semen from the bull and then analyse it on the spot to see if there are the right number of live sperm. Now this may not sound a particularly difficult job, but one thing no one has control of is the bull's desire to perform for you. If you're getting a blood sample you may find it difficult to hold the animal and find a vein, but at worst it's down to a battle of wits between you and the animal. Getting a semen sample, on the other hand, is completely down to whether or not the bull decides to play his part in the affair.

I am not well known for my patience. There are always so many jobs which need doing in the practice that I hate being held up for any reason. I like to arrive at a place, do the job and leave as quickly as possible. So the prospect of standing around all afternoon waiting for a bull to feel the urge did not fill me with enthusiasm.

WHEN I GOT there Davie and Grant were waiting.

'Hello, George. One of your favourite jobs today then!' They were going to enjoy this even if I didn't. I could see that I was going to be the central attraction in this afternoon's work, not the bull. I wouldn't have been surprised if they'd had a bet on how long it would be before I lost my temper. I was equally sure they wouldn't be disappointed.

They had the teaser cow in one side of a barn, and the bull in a pen next door. The idea is that the cow which is bulling, that is on heat, is put in next to the bull to arouse him. Then as he mounts her I interrupt the proceedings with the equipment to collect the semen. It sounds simple enough, I'll agree.

I set up my improvised laboratory in a corner of the barn, on top of an old radiogram which had been dumped there. I carefully lifted my old brass microscope out of the wooden carrying case which is almost as much a work of art as the instrument itself. I've had it since I was a student and I'm very fond of it. Then I got out the rest of the equipment: an artificial vagina. This takes the form of a long Bakelite tube with an inner rubber tube.

Now a further complication is that even if the bull is in the right mood and decides to cooperate, he's very fussy about the temperature of the object he is going to serve into. In nature of course this will be warm and inviting, but the mechanical vagina is made from rubber and is nowhere near as warm as he likes it. So the next stage is to fill the gap between the inner and outer tubes with hot water to warm it up and approach the correct environment for the bull to feel at home. This all has to be done on a cold, windswept day in a corner of a draughty byre.

The boys know the routine so they'd got the kitchen kettle out. They had been joined by a friend of theirs I'd never seen before: obviously the word had gone out that today's turn was going to be from the vet.

EVENTUALLY ALL THE bits and pieces were prepared, and I told the boys, with their permanent grins, to tether the cow and let the bull in. Even though they stood to be told that £3000 worth of their purchased goods were faulty, they were determined not to let that spoil their enjoyment of the afternoon.

Standing next to the cow like a matador in a bull ring awaiting the arrival of his adversary, I heard my opponent leave the outer ring and head towards his arena. Then, horror upon horrors, I looked up and saw over a ton of breeding machine heading at full tilt straight for my precious brass microscope. Forty or so years of bending over looking into its eyepiece, lovingly caressing the well worn handles, passed before my eyes as I prepared to say a fond farewell to it. I imagined picking up the fragments of glass and twisted metal, all that would be left of something that had previously survived being dropped by fellow students, used by my children as a something to stand on to reach top shelves, and accidentally covered with disinfectant by eager young assistants. And here, in this of all situations, it was about to meet an ignominious end. I wondered whether some hand of fate was driving the bull to destroy the instrument by which his destiny would be decided.

Then, just as I had given up hope, the bull veered away and came rushing into the pen. I have never been so pleased to see a bull charging towards me as I was at that moment.

If you think I'm getting increasingly worked up as I recount the events of the day, then you'd be right. Even thinking about the whole process, as I sit writing here in the comfort and warmth of the kitchen, makes me run hot and cold!

I suppose I should have guessed that this was to set the tone of the rest of the afternoon.

One of the most common reasons for a semen collection failing is that the cow won't stand still. So I was relieved to see that this cow was standing quiet as anything, waiting. The bull went straight to her and started sniffing about. For a brief moment I thought that this bovine Casanova would be up within seconds and I wouldn't be ready, so I dashed forwards clutching my contraption in my hands. But it was a false alarm, the bull stood back and looked at me as if to say, 'You're going to have to wait for me on this job, old chap!'

HALF AN HOUR later we were still standing there, numbed by the biting wind blowing right through the barn. The skies had turned thunderously black – like my mood. The enforced inaction was no one's fault but that somehow made it even more vexing because there was no one to vent my anger on. The Nicolson brothers stood as still as the bull and, seemingly, equally unmoved by the whole procedure.

THERE WAS NOTHING else to do really except concentrate attention on that particular part of the anatomy which would force us into action. I tried to calm myself down by thinking about the Nicolsons. They're a great family, strong characters, mentally and physically. Davie and Grant, the two sons with me today, have been known to stick up for their point of view with their fists, and I don't think I'd like to be on the wrong end of their anger.

FOR SOME TIME Davie had been making a clucking noise between his teeth, directed at the bull. I wasn't quite sure whether he was just humming to himself or whether he was trying to speed up the happening with some magic sound. 'Does your wife make that sound to you when she wants you to make love to her, Davie?'

'No, George, but I haven't got any oysters, like she always tempts me with,' came the reply, quick as anything.

'Perhaps we should try the nettles.' Grant's suggestion brought back to me the old farmer's trick of gently rubbing nettles across the bull's testicles. I didn't think that in this case it would be a good idea. The artificial vagina which had been so carefully prepared was becoming colder by the minute. Although I knew that the likelihood of getting any sort of result that afternoon was becoming less, I told the boys to refill the kettle so that we could have another go, and give the bull a change of scenery for a few minutes.

DAVIE LED THE bull around the barn for a while, until I was ready again. It was almost like resuming seats at a theatre after the interval, except that we were all in the play. Standing playing the waiting game again, my mind turned to other members of the Nicolson family. Their sister, Mary Anne, is doing her post-graduate degree in medicine. The parents, Donald and Margaret, run another farm on this Dunphail estate which is owned by Sir Hector Laing, chairman of United Biscuits.

Sir Hector is well liked and respected in the area. A while back Donald Nicolson had a heart condition and I think they'd virtually written him off and said that he'd be dead within six months. Margaret Nicolson must have told Sir Hector because he flew him down to the heart hospital in London in his private jet. They operated on him and he's doing fine now. That to me is a great example of a benefactor to the community, and people respect that sort of person.

Still no sign of action from the bull. . . .

AFTER AN HOUR I decided that I would have to reheat the water again. There we were, three grown men (the stranger had long ago lost interest and departed), standing around completely inactive, waiting for a sign that the bull was about to serve. Still, the concentration had to be maintained. The last time I found myself performing this duty I'd been standing around for ages and my mind had drifted off when all of a sudden there was a movement from the bull. I flung myself forwards without really sorting out in my mind what I was doing, and before I knew it the bull had mounted the cow. I shoved the apparatus up to the bull's erect penis before it could enter the cow, but in the rush I must have missed, because the next I knew there was a warm feeling on my arm and the damn thing had served into my sleeve! It may seem strange but I didn't really mind – at least I managed to get a sample to prove the claim!

However, in this case there was no such indication and I have to say that my patience was nearly worn through. The icy wind had seeped into every bone of my body and sapped what little enthusiasm I might have had. After an hour and a half it was obvious that the bull had no intention of doing anything and I would have to pack up and return another day.

ON THE WAY back home I gradually managed to calm down. The journey back took me across the flat, rough grouse-moors, past the old railway line with the solid-looking stationmaster's house and the stone viaduct which I think is a listed structure now. Looking at all this familiar scenery helped to put the frustrations of the call into perspective, and remind me that of all the times I had driven along that road, very few had been after such a trying afternoon.

Now, sitting here in the warmth of the kitchen, it's quite funny to think of how angry I got. Jane's at the other end of the table working on the accounts and we've been discussing what to charge for this afternoon's call. From a financial point of view it really was a dead loss – I won't be able to charge very much for it. But then we couldn't run our practice on the basis of saying that our time is worth £27.50 an hour and that's what we charge whatever the circumstances. That would mean that in a case like the bull this afternoon I'd have had to charge around £80.

You have to work on a swings and roundabouts system. If we charged the full rate for every job we did, it would simply mean discontent among our clients. It's a two-way relationship, and it would be pointless carrying on if it weren't a fair one both ways. It's really important to get the balance right, so that the farmers knew that they can call us in when there's something wrong with an animal, before it develops into anything serious. If our fees were high, the temptation would be for farmers to leave a problem to see if time and their own efforts could solve it. Then what would happen is that it would get worse and we'd end up getting called to an emergency which needed more drastic treatment or surgery. Or, worse, we wouldn't be called until it was too late to do anything.

Losing an animal is not a satisfactory situation for the farmer from a financial point of view, nor is it professionally satisfying for us. So we operate with as low charges as possible in a deliberate attempt to encourage people to call us in early. And woe betide any who don't do that – they know they'd get an earful from me!

At the end of the day I have to live in the community. I think people's opinion of you is important: you've always got to be aware of your image. It's important for a professional man that the clients think of him as somebody who knows his job, enjoys his work and gives an economic service.

Jane and I have just been talking about this and she remembered one farmer who always used to phone up and say, 'Get the vet to call in when he's passing.' He only did this because he was too mean to pay for a full call-out. Anyway I got so fed up with his attitude that one day I did actually do what he said and called to see him on the way back rather than making him first call. By the time I got there the calf which he'd said wasn't in need of urgent attention was dead. I was so angry that I really shouted at him long and hard about how badly he treated his animals and how he'd have to pull his socks up or find another vet. I was red in the face and really quite shaken by my own anger but as I got in the car to leave he said, 'Well thanks very much. Drive carefully now. Look after yourself.' I felt about three inches tall!

I have to confess that sometimes I'm a bit short on the draw with my temper. Although I have been beaten in that respect by some of my clients. There was one, Donnie, who I called on one day, and he got fiercely angry with me because I'd sent an assistant out to a case rather than going myself, and he'd lost the calf. We stood in the middle of the farmyard in the pouring rain shouting at each other. He screamed at me, 'If you'd bloody come yourself I never would have lost it.' He went on and on, really gave me a hard time.

I shouted back at him, 'I can't be everywhere. It wouldn't have made any difference in any case, I'd have done the same myself.' So there we were, getting more and more heated and all of a sudden he got so annoyed that his eyes crossed in temper! It stopped me completely. I really thought he was going to explode like one of those cartoon characters. I've never seen it happen to anyone else before or since.

I was telling this story to his cousin and he said, 'That's nothing. I saw him get in such a rage one day that he took off his bonnet, threw it on the floor and jumped up and down on it!'

At least this afternoon I'd managed to keep my temper under control.

SUNDAY 19 MARCH

I T'S BEEN ONE OF THOSE DAYS, GEORGE, was Neil
Meldrum's greeting as I opened the car door. 'I had one calved
last night and what a beast. I was down every two hours
during the night checking, but there were a couple I didn't look
at.' There was no mistaking the anger directed at himself. 'One
was round the back and she must have been going for a while
when I found her. I got the calf out but damn it, I was too late
and it was dead.'

Just like a pregnant woman's, a cow's waters break and it
lies down and starts pushing. As long as it's found it can be helped,
but last night's was one Neil had missed. There was no disguising
the despondency in his voice. 'I skinned the calf and put it on one
of the bought in calves, George.' Farmers buy extra calves so that
if a cow loses its own calf it can be persuaded to foster another.

I'd been called in to attend another cow which had started
calving just a while ago. In these situations I feel even more
desperate to achieve positive results. From the details Neil had
given to Jane on the phone just half an hour or so earlier it had
sounded like it would have to be a caesarean section, a prospect
which I still find exciting from a professional point of view.

'She's in the barn with another which calved last night,
George, and I've got your spotlight fixed up.' This was a comment
on all the moaning that had gone on last time I went to a case
there and found that I could hardly see my hand, let alone
anything as fine as the scalpel!

While Neil had been talking I'd got my bag from the boot of
the car. I'd been on a routine blood testing call to a farm about
15 miles away, which is why I always carry all the instruments I
might need for a caesarean section in the car with me everywhere.
The practice is so spread out, we might be 30 miles away from
home and get a call to travel another 10 miles to a case. It's no
use having to go back home to pick up the stuff and then go out
again, so the instruments are always kept in a sterilised bag in
the back of the car. As soon as I get home the instruments are
put on top of the stove and boiled up again ready for the next
time they're needed.

Neil led the way into the barn where the black-and-white cow stood alongside some rails which divided the barn in half. On the other side fifty or so sheep looked on. 'Are they for fattening, Neil?'

'Yes, I'm feeding them on pellets.'

'No hay or anything?'

'No, just pure pellets to fatten them up quickly so that I can catch the height of the market.' The farming system tends to split into those farmers who specialise in breeding animals and others who buy them to fatten up for slaughter.

'Is it going to be a good year, Neil?' I asked, knowing what the reply would be.

'You should know better than to ask a farmer that question, George!' At least some of the tension in Neil's face had lifted now.

As I set out the instruments on the table which Neil had placed in the middle of the barn, two shafts of unseasonally warm, late afternoon sunlight came streaming through the window at the end of the barn and the skylight overhead, overcoming years of cobwebs and dust. The sunlight cast a golden glow on the straw which covered the floor of the barn. The scene was almost biblical, all we needed was another wise man!

Looking at the size of the cow I could see that she had a large calf inside her. It's the usual problem, caused by crossing heifers with large continental bulls – in this case, Neil told me, a Charolais. The farmers get better prices for the calves, as long as we get them out alive, which is why we're doing more caesarean sections when we get to them in time. 'I was over at Glenlivet the other day, Neil, where they've got that herd of pedigree Charolais.' I talked as I poured warm water into the instrument bowl. 'Do you know they are so big inside that my arms were hardly long enough to manipulate the calf. I think if they're going to breed such big cows in the future they'll have to breed veterinary surgeons with bigger arms as well!' Neil helped me on with the calving gown.

Usually Neil's wife Dodo would have come out to assist at the operation. I like to get the farmer's wives to help because they've usually got the cleanest hands on the farm!

'She's not been well, George, so you'll have to put up with my wee hands!'

I looked at the two great hands which were tying the halter on to the cow. 'Well, let's hope we don't need to do any micro-surgery then! And for God's sake wash them before we do anything.' I have a bee in my bonnet about hygiene. Most post-

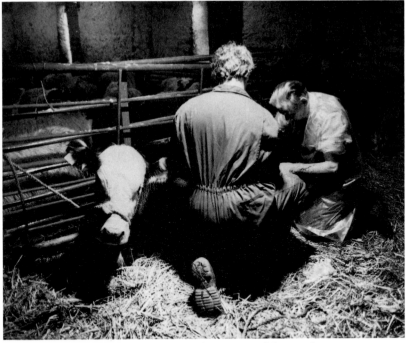

Neil Meldrum assists me in sewing up after a successful operation.

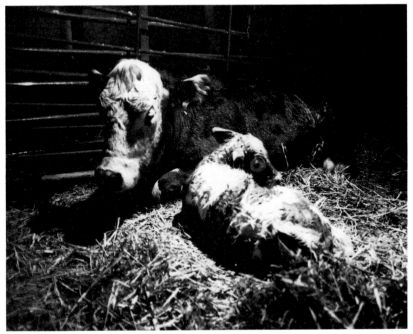

Mother and child doing well.

operative problems come from infections which are caused while an animal's opened up. It's relatively easy when you're in the stainless steel environment of a hospital theatre to keep everything sterilised, but when your nurse also has to pull on the rope from time to time to keep the beast up, or heave an animal's backside around to make it possible to operate on, it's not quite so easy. I'm sure that the boys get fed up with me nagging them about washing their hands every time they touch anything which might not be clean, but I'd rather nag than risk infection.

I would normally have given the cow a full internal examination but I could see from her size that she wasn't going to be able to calve normally, and I didn't want to dirty my hands and risk infection. Besides, Neil had calved enough from the same bull to know when there were likely to be problems, and he was convinced as well that a caesarean was called for. After his fatality of the night I didn't want him to have any more.

The cow was standing, tied to the dividing rail, and the sheep started to line up for a view on the other side. It reminded me of the people you see on television at the last night of the proms pressing in behind the conductor.

The first step is to give the cow an injection of sedative to quieten her down, then disinfect the skin and inject a local anaesthetic along the line the cut will take. While both drugs are taking effect I shave the area around where the cut will go.

'When you retire, George, you can always set up a fancy hairdressing place in Grantown.' Neil was definitely sounding a bit more cheerful.

Having shaved the line of the cut I took the scalpel and gently made the first incision through the skin. Then deeper again through the three layers of muscle, gradually deepening the cut. Then through the peritoneum, a thin layer of white skin which lies between the muscle and the inside of the abdomen. This part has to be done carefully because if you cut too far you might nick the stomach.

When I had made the final cut I was suddenly aware of a strange crunching sound behind my right ear, which I'd previously been oblivious to in my state of concentration. I looked in the direction of the sound and saw a small face only a few feet away from me, staring intently at the innards which were unfolding before it.

It was Wayne, Neil's five-year-old son, standing motionless,

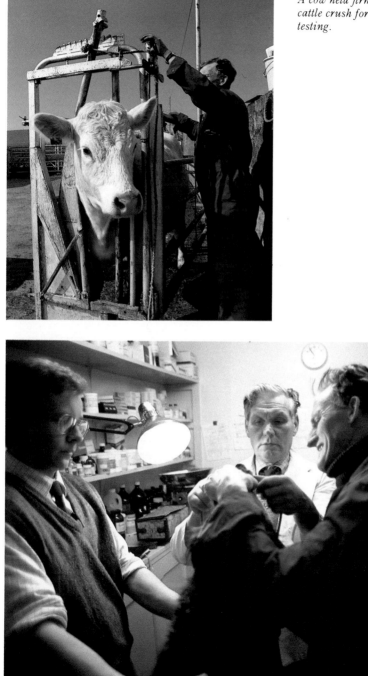

A cow held firmly in the cattle crush for TB testing.

The examination which revealed cancer in Bill and Florence's dog.

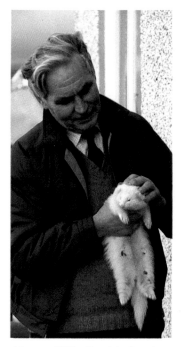

Above *'Miss Ferrie', the mis-
sexed ferret, returning to his
owner.*

Right *At the height of calving
much of my time is spent in byres
like this.*

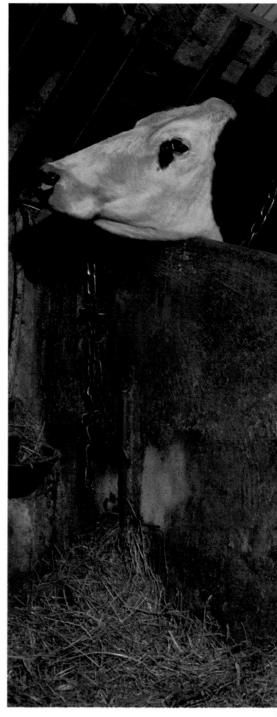

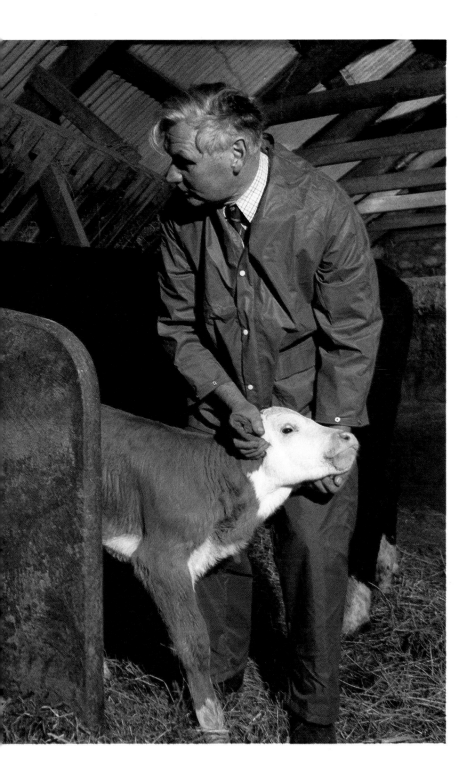

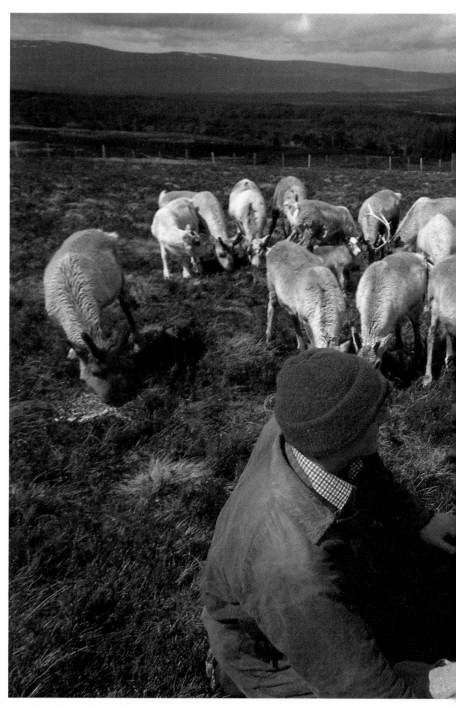

Alan Smith and I examine a reindeer calf, high up on the Cairngorms.

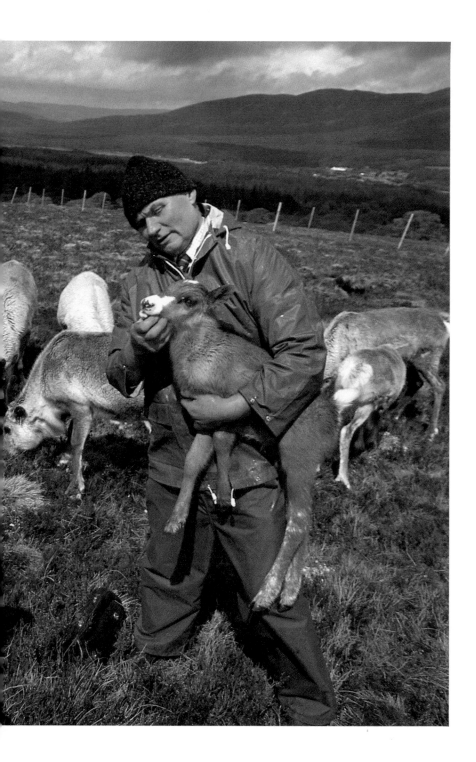

Dawn mist in the valley below the Cromdale Hills.

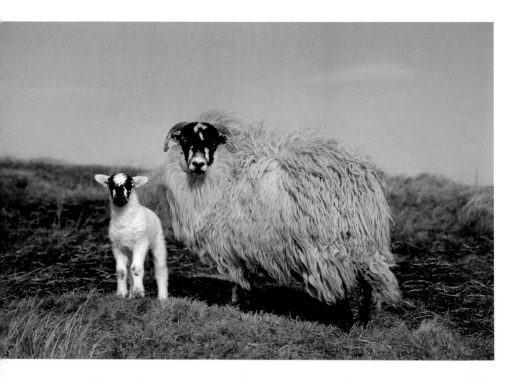

Above *Black-faced ewe with her lamb.*

Right *Well-earned hospitality after a day's work in the fields – tea, cake and a wee dram in the warmth of the farm kitchen.*

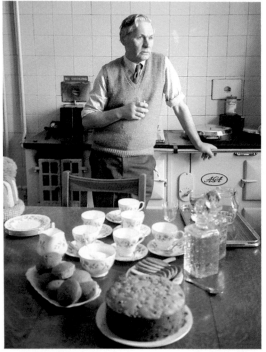

except for the chomping jaw, one hand holding a crisp packet, the other deep inside it ready to supply the next mouthful. Alongside him stood his younger brother, Mark. Both were wearing miniature versions of the overalls worn by Dad.

The cow's stomach fell sideways out of the incision at this stage of the proceedings, so that I could get my hand in behind to feel the uterus.

As I leant against the cow to delve inside, I saw that the audience were really being held by the performance and couldn't wait for the second act. Glancing from Neil to the boys, I could see great similarities. No sign of any emotion in any of them, just intense concentration. Here were two embryonic farmers if ever I saw them.

The cow was doing well. She stood patiently as we worked on the cut in her side. I pushed my hand into the incision and as my hand slipped gently around the womb I could clearly feel the features of the creature waiting to be let into the world. My mind built up such a vivid picture from the impression gained by my hands, that I could almost imagine the calf stretching its head to lick my fingers. I was relieved to feel that it was in the correct position to pull it out.

The next stage was to move the uterus so that I could make another incision, this time through the uterus wall. Then the magic moment that I never tire of. Through the gap made by the cut I felt for the hind legs. Then, gently at first, I lifted out the calf. I'm sure it must look like a conjurer pulling a rabbit out of a hat.

I wasn't expecting a round of applause but equally nor was I expecting the question from Wayne, 'Why did it come out of its belly and not its bum, Dad?'

However this was not really the time for a full explanation of the whys and wherefores of caesarean sections – more important at this moment was the patient.

'Right, Neil, hold the legs and swing.' There was really no need to tell him what to do. We swung the calf a few times to remove anything in its mouth and airways.

The calf gave a few coughs and shook its head, so we knew that all was well with it. The final part of the operation was to stitch the cow up again. At this stage the cow has her stomach hanging out and part of the uterus showing, and stage by stage I pieced it back together again. The boys had gone to look at the new calf which was already showing signs of movement, but were back now looking at the open wound on the cow. They stood very still again, Wayne only moving to put another crisp in his mouth or absentmindedly offer one to his brother.

I often say to a farmer that it's a good sign if the calf gets up and knocks the table over, and sure enough this newly born creature was already taking a few teetering steps towards its mother, who we were still working on. Then came the crash. It must have heard me and had moved under the table, tried to stand up and literally knocked it over. I couldn't feel anger because it was such a good sign of health that it really didn't matter.

'Dad?' piped up a small voice. 'Is there going to be any more blood?' Neil explained that now all the innards had been sewn back in place, there wouldn't be. The show lost its appeal immediately and the two boys wandered off in search of other forms of entertainment.

I went out to check on a couple of other calves that were only a day old and then went back into the barn to pick up my bag of instruments.

It never ceased to amaze me that within half an hour of being born the calf was walking, albeit inelegantly, towards its mother who then licked it all over. In the old days before we were really into doing caesars we would have tried to calve that cow, and the calf, and possibly the heifer, would have died. At best she would have been pushed around a hell of a lot and been in a lot of pain. With this operation she was stitched up and looking pretty proud of herself and the new addition to her family.

And when I left the farm Neil had a smile on his face.

WEDNESDAY 29 MARCH

I SHOT IT YESTERDAY AFTERNOON, explained Gary, a young lad who's chief ranger at the Highland Wildlife Park. He opened the door to the post-mortem room to reveal the carcass of a red deer calf lying on the floor. 'It was on its last legs, George, and being knocked about by the Highland cattle and the stags.'

'Well, you did right to put it out of its misery, Gary.' My first reaction to the sight of the deer carcass which lay before us on the post-mortem room floor was that it was pretty emaciated. We turned the carcass on its back so that I could start to open it up, and were joined by Jeremy, the parks curator. 'This is the third calf that's got so thin, George,' he said, 'and there are two more which look as though they're on the way out.'

We're lucky that the PM room isn't used very often at the park, but it's very handy when it is needed. It's a stark room with a concave floor sloping towards a drain in the centre. This helps to stop the place from becoming awash with blood. As we turned the carcass over I could see that there were no lice on it, often a cause of poor condition. There were signs of bruising, probably from where it had been knocked about by the other animals. I opened up the body and started to go through the various organs. One of the common causes of death is puncture of the lung by another stag's antlers, but I could tell that wasn't the case here. These lungs and heart were in first class condition, nice and pink and soft.

'Let's take out what the gamekeepers euphemistically call the green offal,' I said. The stomach and bowels came out and it started to pong a bit. It's not a smell I mind too much; the only smell I could never stand was babies' nappies. Thank goodness I had an understanding wife who never asked me to change one. I don't think I could have managed it!

The deer was so thin that it was pretty obvious something serious had caused it to lose condition. In sheep we would probably suspect liver fluke, but red deer are seldom affected by it. There was certainly no sign of that here; the liver was clean and healthy. There was a well-documented outbreak of liver fluke in the mid-1930s in the north-west of Scotland when thousands upon thousands of sheep died, and yet no deaths were recorded among the red deer.

I carried on the rest of the examination and there was no sign of anything else in the intestines. But I suspected that minute intestinal worms were to blame. It's not just been the skiers who've had problems with this year's warm winter; the animals have as well. Normally the worms become dormant with the cold weather, but it's been so mild that they've been crawling up through the ground and the larvae have been hatching out. Then they sitting on top of the grass where the sheep in particular eat them. I think it's probably the same for the deer, so I took a sample of the faeces which I must look at later on tonight.

JEREMY ASKED ME if I could have a look at the sea eagles before I left. The park has two which were recently imported from Stockholm. They've been in quarantine for thirty days, so they only have five days to go before their time is up. We made our way in through the outer wire door of the isolation aviary and closed it behind us. It's second nature to these zoo people to close one door before they open another.

In the first of the two cages was a beautiful grey bird of prey. It stood on its perch, about 2 feet tall, cocking its head to one side, and all the time keeping its eyes on us. It looked fierce and forbidding, rather like an old schoolteacher I used to have. I was glad that I didn't have to take a blood sample off it, though this one has a bent, deformed claw, probably as a result of being caught in a trap, so maybe it wouldn't be able to do too much damage.

It was originally Russian, from Moscow zoo, and was sent to Stockholm zoo as part of a breeding programme – they wanted a male to replace one that had died. They were a bit upset, and there were a few red faces, when it was discovered that it was a female. In all species of birds of prey the female is considerably larger than the male – I suppose that's what being hen-pecked is all about – so it's a bit difficult to imagine how the error was made.

The second cage holds a male sea eagle which was illegally caught in Norway, and hand reared. He won't be able to be released because he's actually imprinted himself on to human beings, and relates more to us than to his peers. I have fed him from my hand, he's so tame. It's quite a frightening sight, this great bird heading towards you. You always hope that it's read its cookery book and realises that it wouldn't really like the taste of your hand!

THE LAST PATIENT at the Wildlife Park today was in the guest bedroom at Jeremy's house in the grounds of the Wildlife Park. Jeremy lifted the lid on a wooden box in the corner and removed a small, black, sleek creature. The baby otter cub has been staying as a guest for the last couple of weeks. It was washed out from its holt when it was about six weeks old and brought into the park by the SSPCA (the Scottish version of the RSPCA). The Rothie-murchus estate is donating fish for her from their trout farm. I wanted to give her a distemper vaccine now that she'd be mixing with other animals.

I explained to Jeremy that I haven't a great deal of experience of vaccinating otters, but dogs are usually a bit upset afterwards, and sometimes a bit off their food.

'Well, they're called dog and bitch, otters,' explained Jeremy. 'Although she's a bit of a cross between a puppy and a kitten in her antics sometimes.' And sure enough as Jeremy put her down on the floor she started to dart around mischievously, running between our feet and over our shoes. 'Since she's been on meat she seems far more active,' he said as we watched the antics on the floor. 'It's obviously part of her development.'

Jeremy warmed to his subject. 'At this age her eyesight's pretty poor, though I don't think they have very good sight at the best of times. But their hearing's good despite having these tiny ears, and their sense of smell is very acute.'

The otter was quite an endearing little thing with her tiny paws, bright eyes and sharp teeth. Great for catching eels, I should think. Jeremy's children joined us and were obviously well used to having the otter about the house. It seemed to recognise the daughter Rosemary, ran over towards her and was soon in her arms.

'Have you decided on a name for her yet?' I asked Rosemary. She looked thoughtful and shook her head.

'It'll have to be something Scottish like Bonnie Mary,' I said.

That's one of the things I really enjoy about making calls at the Wildlife Park. There's quite often an unusual animal to treat and it's great to be able to learn something new and be taxed a bit in your work. It certainly stops you getting complacent.

TUESDAY 11 APRIL

I HAVEN'T BEEN keeping up with the diary for a while because we've been so busy every minute of the day and night. I'm sure most people's idea of spring is a beautiful, gentle time of year when the flowers are blossoming and the lambs are gambolling in the fields and all is well with the world. In farming circles the reality is often very far from that ideal, and it can be the worst time of year. Most farmers are calving and lambing and that takes a heck of a lot of effort and time. It usually coincides with the first opportunity to get out and work in the fields, and it's very difficult for a farmer to stay inside with the cows and ewes, even when there's plenty to do there, when he also knows that he should be out making the best of every minute of good weather. The animals are often at their lowest in terms of condition, because they've used up their reserves during the cold of the winter. It's just like us, when we get run down we take a cold a lot easier.

Even though the weather has been pretty kind to us over the last few months, we still seem to have suffered. In particular from an incredibly virulent strain of bug which has been causing scour, a sort of dysentery, in young calves. We've four farms that have been hit by it very badly, and I'm at a bit of a loss to know what to try next. I've sent off numerous samples to the labs but so far they've reported negative, with no sign of any virus. But I know damn well that there's something there. I've been out to the farms every day for a few days now, and, if anything, the calves seem to be getting worse. If I'm not careful the farmers will get fed up with us making return calls, and become disgruntled. They say, 'The vet's been here and keeps coming back and yet there's no sign of improvement.' Because it's their busy time of year a lot of them get very depressed about the situation, so we have to be psychologists as well as vets. Part of our job is to listen to their complaints and reassure them that everything will turn out all right. It's no use going in with a long face – you've got to be cheerful.

The farmers I feel sorry for are the single men. There's one person in particular who had a calf that just died on us. If he had a wife he could have gone in and said 'that bloody calf died' and

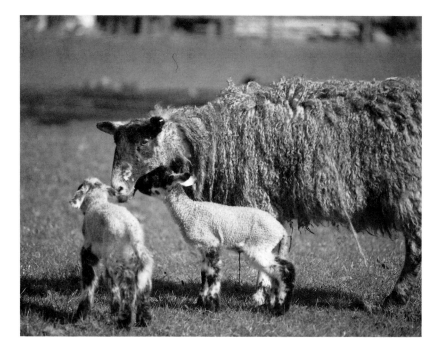

got some support from her. But he has no one to share the load. That must be pretty miserable, especially at a time of year like this when calves seem to be taking ill a lot.

I've had my fill of these chronic cases today; it gets really depressing. One farmer has got cattle down with the scour, and a couple of other bad cases. Another has a calf with pneumonia, a third has a calf just wasting away and I haven't got a clue what's up with it. Willie and Neil have both been to see it but neither achieved anything and left it in mid-air, which is where the boss gets the job of picking up the pieces. I suppose it's quite understandable really – it's easier for me to be bold and try a drastic cure than it is for them. It's something they'll have to learn, though. So today I told the farmer, George McConachie, that I'll open up the wasted calf tomorrow to see if there's a stone or something lodged in its innards which is stopping it eating. That really is a long shot, and to be truthful it will just be pot luck as to whether we find anything or not. But the farmer's happier: he knows that we're doing something, and it makes the case more positive in his mind. If it dies under the anaesthetic or the day after, I'll not be happy but at least we'll have tried something. The farmer won't mind because he'll feel we've tried,

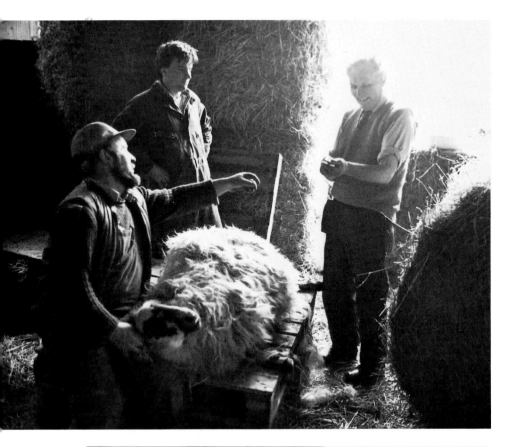

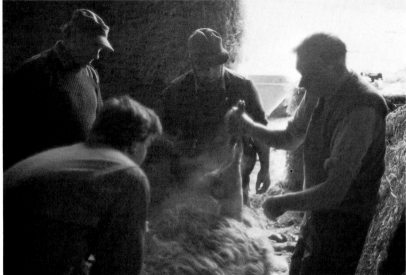

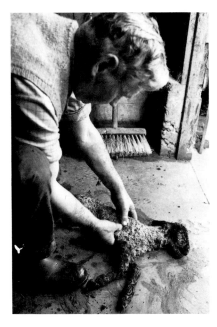

A caesarean on a ewe.
Far left above *Preparing the anaesthetic before the incision.*
Far left below *Pulling out the first lamb.*
Left *Resuscitating the second lamb.*
Below *A few moments later the twins are almost on their feet.*

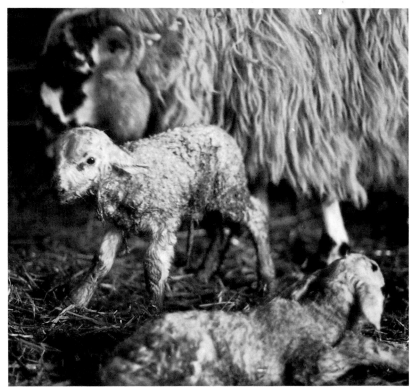

and of course if we find something then everyone will be happy. There's nothing these people hate more than inaction on anyone's part.

While I was there I had to have a look at a heifer which he'd bought to fatten up and sell for meat. He reckons it's pregnant which would mean that he'd lose out on profits from selling her, and have an extra calf to look after. There are set rules laid down for this sort of case. He will have to report it to the auctioneer who'll go back to the seller and then he has a choice of selling it back for the original price plus something for the cost of keeping it, or hanging on to it until it has calved and taking the risk that he might lose it. We put the animal in a cattle crush outside, and sure enough she was about eight months pregnant. So they'll have to sort it all out pretty quickly within the next month.

The only respite from all these depressing calls was that at one of the farms I had to give a hand at a lambing. We were just walking back to the car through one of the huge lambing sheds, sort of delivery wards, when Stuart, the farmer, saw that one of the ewes was having problems. When we went over to her, we saw that she had already given birth to one live lamb. She was licking it into life even as she was panting away trying to bring the second lamb into the world. The other twenty or so ewes in that area cleared a space for us to work, and stood in the far corner of the pen chewing the straw and taking no more than a passing interest in what we were up to.

These sheds are the modern way of lambing and calving. They make things easier for the farmer – he can keep an eye on a large flock twenty-four hours a day. Stuart's got about seven hundred sheep, and he was telling me that he had thirty ewes give birth during the day yesterday, which is going some. Most of them will be twins or triplets, and that's a lot of lambs. Stuart was keeping pretty cheerful considering he'll be working solidly from five in the morning until gone eleven at night at the moment. It's easy to see how farmers can get depressed, though, when they've suddenly got to nurse a dozen or so sick calves on top of everything else. Stuart's lucky, he has a great wee wife, Elsie, who looks after the newly born lambs, and bottle-feeds any that need help. Last year at one time she was bottle-feeding seventy orphaned lambs as well as looking after the maternity needs of the rest of the flock, and cooking and generally running the house. I can always tell when she's really harassed, because she ties her hair up in a bun on top of her head with baler twine.

If I hadn't been there Stuart and Elsie would have managed this morning's case with no problem, but I really enjoy births so I didn't need too much persuading to help out.

As we moved towards the ewe, she took off, so we flung ourselves at her, managing to grab her fleece. As I soaped my arm Stuart held up the rear legs so that I could reach into the ewe. Sure enough, the lamb's head was twisted, which was why it was having problems popping out. I manipulated the body and grabbed hold of the legs. The lamb came out smoothly and I swung it around my head to remove any of the fluids from its mouth, then laid it on the straw in front of mum.

'I'll just feel inside to see if she's all right,' I said to Stuart as he moved the two lambs together. To my delight I felt that she held a surprise inside. 'There's another one in here, Stuart.'

Stuart held up the ewe's hind legs again and I reached further inside. Like a conjurer performing his favourite trick, I produced a third lamb and swung it in the air around my head. By the time I left, the three new additions were already cleaned up, had taken their first uncertain steps, and were sucking away at the mother. The exhilaration of acting as a midwife was a bit of light relief in what had otherwise been a dour day.

WHEN I GOT back to the surgery Willie was just finishing off a caesarian section on a ewe. We carry out more and more caesars like this as the years go by. Usually the farmers bring them to us and we use the garage as an operating theatre. We've done four between us over the last few days, some of them with live lambs, others where we've had to open them up to get dead bodies out. Judging by the plaintive bleating coming from the garage, this one had a successful outcome.

THE SURGERY BROUGHT another case of a working dog which is on its way out. You feel sad when any dog proves to be suffering from an incurable disease, but when it's a good working dog it's even worse. Michael's face was grave as he held his black-and-white collie. It had lumps all over its body and I had to tell him that it had leukaemia, and that sadly it really wouldn't be around for long. The only thing I could do was to give it some pills and an injection. They won't provide a cure, but they will slow the spread of the illness, and hopefully reduce the size of the lumps.

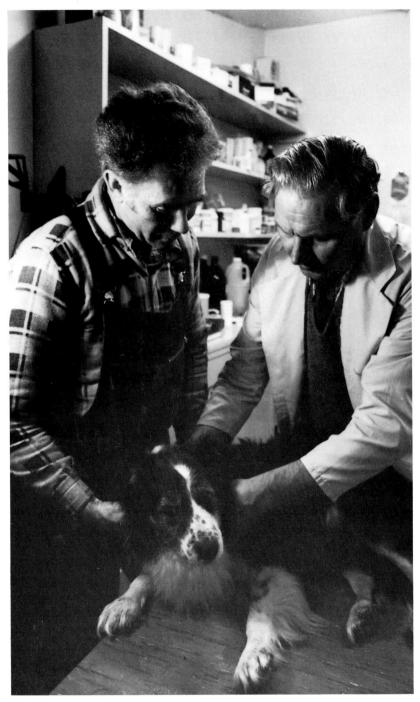

Examining Michael's collie in the surgery.

'I want to find a new dog, George, before this one goes.' Michael rubbed his forehead with his strong hands as he spoke. We travel around so much that we hear about new litters, and we can often solve two people's problems at once.

I had a sudden flash of inspiration. 'You're looking for a new dog. Would you mind going up to Donnie Ross and dropping off some pills for him?' I'd heard that he had some collie pups and by coincidence his wife had phoned earlier asking for medicines, but we hadn't been down that way today. Michael could do us a favour in return for the information about the pups, which he willingly did. That's the great thing about living in such a close community.

Neil was amused when another dog came in with warts, and I told him to try the old fashioned method of tying a piece of thin cotton around it very tightly. With any luck the wart will just drop off after a few days. It wasn't worth operating on so it was either that or charm it away, and I'm a bit low on witchcraft at the moment. The dog had come in for an injection to stop her coming on heat. 'If it wasn't for sex we'd be out of work!' I said to her owner as she left.

After tidying up the surgery, Willie, Neil and I sat in the kitchen writing up our record books. It's a good time of day to discuss the problems we've encountered and any treatments we've given which may be out of the ordinary. I posed an ethical question for debate. 'I had a farmer today who told me that he was going to buy in some lambs from a particular other farm. I know that the second farmer has enzootic abortion rife in his flock. What should I have done?'

It's one of those problems which doctors face increasingly with AIDS, whether to pass on information to another person who might be fatally affected. With this enzootic abortion a healthy flock could catch it from an incoming animal and the next set of lambs could be lost.

Willie and Neil thought about the problem. The dilemma was that if I didn't say anything the first farmer could go ahead and buy a lamb which could then infect the rest of his flock and ruin him. On the other hand if I did tell him not to buy because I knew that the other farmer's flock was infected I would be breaking all the rules of confidentiality. In a small community like ours the news would soon spread and the second farmer would then have difficulty in selling any of his flock, even when they were all clear.

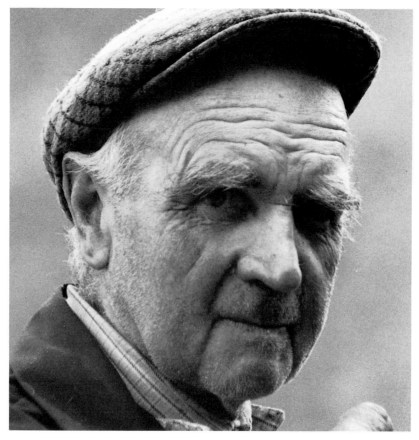

Duncan Durno

At the end of our discussion, I told Willie and Neil what I *had* done. I'd decided that the middle course was the best one, so I'd suggested to the first farmer that it was a heck of a long way to go to buy a lamb and that he could probably buy one nearer home. That was all I could do, really, and I hope that he took the hint. These sorts of problems have no textbook answers; you just have to use common sense, and try to supply a solution which is best for all parties. It's really important to think hard when you're faced with a problem like this, and make the right decision; a thoughtless decision either way could harm a lot of people.

AFTER THE BOYS had left Jane and I were sitting in the kitchen doing the books when we had another caller, Duncan Durno, one of the luminaries of the farming world in Strathspey. He'd come in to pick up some drugs, and as usually happens on these occasions we sat down and had a general chat about what's going on in the district. I was telling him about the terrible problems I've been having with scour, and that I was tearing my hair out trying to work out what was wrong with the calves. Without a moment's hesitation he supplied the answer. 'Two pounds of barley,' he said with great authority. 'That will sort it out.'

Duncan is the very epitome of a good farmer. He and his sons know their stock and how to look after their animals. You go to operate on things there and they recover and thrive. I reckon you could cut an animal's head off on their farm and it would survive. You know that when they're beside you, everything will go to plan. If you say to them, 'Hold that tail,' you can be confident that the tail would come off before they'd let go. That sort of professionalism really helps the vet in his job, and you can be sure that they'll look after the animal properly after you've done your work.

There are some farms where animals with even the most simple complaints never get better, and it's all down to the management of the place. Some people have got the skills required to run a farm, others just haven't and will never acquire them. Duncan and his sons breed champion cattle; he's just won another top prize at one of the shows with one of his beasts, and he's really well respected in the district. It's great that all the efforts of modern drugs and laboratory tests had been able to do nothing, but he was convinced that the cure was quite simple. I'll go to bed now, happy in the knowledge that I've been given the secret of the cure, but frustrated too, that the elusive solution was so simple!

WEDNESDAY 12 APRIL

WHEN I WENT back to Stuart and the other problem farms today to see how they were all getting on, I told them about Duncan's guaranteed barley cure. If anyone else had offered that solution they would all have laughed and dismissed it as a joke. However, because it had come from Duncan they listened intently, being sure to maintain the outward appearance of finding the idea mildly amusing. If I go back tomorrow, I wouldn't be surprised to see a few bags of barley lying around! I hope they won't need it, though, because the good news today was that the calves are getting better. My treatment seems to have been working, but just taking longer than normal because they'd all been affected so badly. Of course if any of the farmers try Duncan's cure it will probably seem as though the barley remedy has done the trick, and I know where the credit for success will lie!

I also operated on the calf with the mystery illness, and discovered that it had a stomach ulcer, the only one I've ever seen in a live animal. So that proved two things: first, my decision that it was better to try kill-or-cure treatment was right, even though I hadn't been sure what I was looking for. Second, even an old boy like me can still learn after forty years in the business. So perhaps after a few weeks of bad times, things are looking up again.

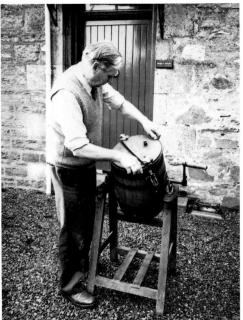

Our antiquated milk churn, donated by a local farmer, used for our equally antiquated method of mixing our drugs. I don't think many vets do this any more.

MONDAY 17 APRIL

AGOOD DEAL of our surgery work tends to be vaccinations and run of the mill cases, but I suppose most nights we get something which requires all our skill and experience. Often it's not so much on the veterinary side as the human psychology aspect of our profession. Tonight Bill and Florence came in with their collie dog and I had a feeling something was not quite right as soon as I saw her.

'When I touched her tonight she winced, you know, George?' Bill said, gently stroking the dog's head.

I started to go through the routine. 'Is she drinking much?'

'I haven't really noticed, George.' His matter-of-fact tone belied the concern which his face expressed. 'She was hurt about five years ago and she lost the use of her tail, but it's back again.'

I saw that there was a lump in her throat and suspected the worst. Bill noticed where I was concentrating my attention. We lifted the dog on to the table; she was certainly thin. 'It's terrible to see her pining away like this,' said Florence,

I called for Neil to come in, and introduced him to Bill and Florence. Then I got Neil to hold the dog while I examined her. Florence looked on intently, biting her nails. 'I noticed that her breath is bad, George,' she said as I pulled the light over the dog and looked into the throat. Sure enough, there was a cancerous growth which started in the tonsils and was spreading through the whole throat, gradually closing it up and making it increasingly difficult for the dog to drink and eat.

'I should have got you to do it last time you were down at the farm, George.' Bill's voice was weary, not a callous response, but a heartfelt one. 'You always want to leave it as long as possible before doing anything about it, don't you? But I can't see her suffering like this any more.' The wife had started to cry so I took her through to the kitchen where Jane got her a drink.

When I got back to the surgery Bill was talking with Neil. 'She was a good dog in her day, working with sheep and cattle,' he said, holding her ear affectionately. 'This will be the last one. I don't need a dog now that I'm not among the cattle.'

He turned to me as I loaded the syringe with Euthatol. 'You always feel sad when you put down a dog, but even worse when it's been a good working dog,' I said.

'In the last couple of years she's been in retirement and more with the wife, so she's taking it harder than me, George,' he replied, as if to explain why he was apparently unmoved. He paused for a few moments, then went on: 'When you see a dog as nice as that suffering, and you can just put it down so gently as that ... why don't they do it to human beings when they have no chance of surviving?'

It's a point of view often expressed by my clients and I must say I have some sympathy with it. Bill stepped back to stand against the wall as I clipped the dog's leg. 'The last one we had was about eight years old and we took her out for a walk one night and she just disappeared. We thought she was chasing rabbits, but I found her later that night. She'd fallen down an old well in the garden which was full of icy water and she'd been scrabbling to try and reach over the edge but couldn't. So she died, and we said, never again. Then we bought another terrier and that one's getting old so it will be the last one definitely.' I thought to myself that I'd heard that before.

I found the vein and prepared to put the needle in. 'Come and see how easy she goes down, Bill,' I said.

Bill just turned his head away: 'I've seen it enough in cattle, George. I know how nicely they go down.' Even though he's a tough old farm worker he couldn't watch his dog in its last moments.

The deed done, Neil brought in a plastic bag and we put the body in it, and took it around the back of the house. Mr Murphy will collect it next time he calls. He disposes of our failures.

Bill was the last person in the surgery, so we went through and joined Florence in the kitchen. She and Jane were talking. She was obviously still upset but eventually we tried to take her mind off things by talking about the big news in the district. Bill's boss, Sandy Innes, had had a burglary at his home in Nairn and his wife Jackie's pearl necklace had been stolen, along with an engagement ring and some other bits and pieces. I remembered where the necklace had come from.

Every year a group of tinkers, called MacMillan I think, would camp out in Cromdale, a village just up the road from us. They came in search of freshwater pearls in the River Spey. They used buckets with glass bottoms in them to look down into the water, and you'd see them there up to their waists in the freezing water looking for mussels for hours on end. I used to think they were mad but judging by the price the pearls are now commanding the only insane thing they did was sell them.

They were boys for the booze and they would go up to Seafield Lodge Hotel which Jackie's mother, Tottie, ran, to try and sell the pearls to get money for drinking. Tottie would buy them very cheaply, but the Macmillan lads were happy to take whatever price they could get. There weren't really many people who were interested in freshwater pearls then, but over the years Tottie must have collected quite a lot. Eventually there were enough to make into a necklace about 4 feet long. 'They say it was worth about £20,000,' said Florence. I'm sure that's right, Strathspey pearls would be worth quite a bit simply for their rarity value. They reckon that for that reason the thief will probably have thrown them away, knowing that he wouldn't be able to sell them – which is even more upsetting.

AFTER BILL AND Florence had gone I couldn't help thinking about another family pet I'd put down many years ago.

It was when my son Andrew was quite small, and a lady came into the surgery with an old but much-loved animal. It was very ill and I said to her that it would be best to put it out of its misery. This started off floods of tears, with her questioning whether it was the right thing to do or not. I talked to her for ages, explaining that it really was going to be better for her pet, and that it was the kindest and most caring thing she could do for it. Eventually she calmed down and was just coming round to the idea, when the door burst open and in came my young son Andrew who must have been three or four then. He stood with his hands in his pockets, looked at what was going on, and summed up the situation by saying, 'Are you going to bump it off, Dad?' Of course this produced a new flood of tears and it took quite a long time before I managed to calm her so that I could do what had to be done. Now that Andrew's a vet himself I hope he's learned a better bedside manner than he exhibited then!

WE HAVE FOUR children, two boys and two girls. They've all done quite well for themselves. The eldest, John, is a solicitor in Edinburgh. Then there's Jean who was a secretary before she married Bill, who's Managing Director of part of the Racal group of companies near Edinburgh. Andrew's next: he's married with

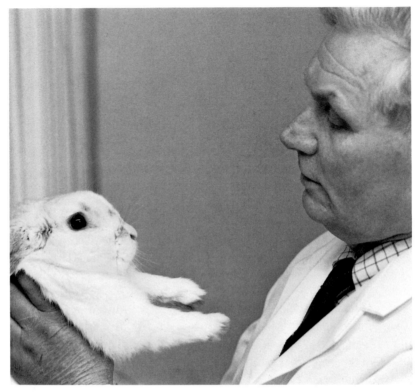

Eye to eye with a patient.

two children, and his veterinary practice is down in Castle Douglas. The youngest is Anne, who married John, a farmer in a neighbouring village, and they have two children. So I'm very lucky that they're all still in Scotland and all have very happy family lives.

That's all thanks to Jane. She brought them up single-handed, with a little help from the farmers' wives. When we had the family I was so busy in the practice that I hardly ever saw them, until they were old enough to take out in the car with me on my rounds. This was before they went to school but after they were house trained and past the nappy stage. When they were really small they'd go into the farm kitchen and the farmers' wives would look after them. Later on I would put them on top of the hayrack, where they'd be safely out of way, but still be able to watch father being knocked about, or knocking about something.

The great thing was that it taught them patience. The children were brought up that the practice was the most important thing. If we were planning to go somewhere and an emergency came in, everything would be cancelled and we'd go to the urgent case. I think that's why they've developed into such reasonable people – because they understood that there were things more important than them, and they weren't king pins.

One day I took Anne to a calving case at Achnahannet – a pedigree Aberdeen Angus heifer, a young cow. When I arrived she was in a long loose box. At one end there was a stable door, the kind in two halves so that you can open the top and keep the bottom half shut for the animal to look out without fear of it getting out. Well, we went in and the farmer and his son were there; the animal was up at the other end. We got ropes on to the calf's legs and the three of us started pulling to get it out. Anne, who was about four then, came over to give a hand and started pulling as well. And that's great because it's good that they want to help even at that age.

We got the calf out alive, cleared the airways and all was well. The heifer was exhausted and she lay there not moving. Anne had wandered off to the far end of the box near the stable door which had the bottom half shut. Suddenly the heifer got up and looked around the barn, settling her gaze on Anne. I could see what was about to happen but there wasn't much I could do. The heifer put her head down and charged her. We had to just watch in horror, and hope. The heifer got to Anne, pushed her head under her and tossed her up over the bottom half of the stable door and out on to the cobble stones. By the time I'd run down towards the door a small head peeped over the top, looking dazed. Luckily she was pretty tough and she wasn't any the worse for it, but it gave us a fright and she never forgot it.

FRIDAY 28 APRIL

BY EIGHT THIRTY this morning I had everything worked out for the day, but as often happens, a call came in from one of the farmers out towards the Glenlivet part of the district. He had a cow that had been calving since just before five thirty in the morning. It had looked as though it was all going smoothly until the calf appeared. It was oversize, had got stuck half way out and died. We treat this as an emergency because the cow is left in a great deal of pain. The only thing to do is to cut the calf up and get it out of the cow piece by piece. The procedure sounds more gruesome than it actually is. It's not a very pleasant job, but certainly one of the more valuable. We can really do some good and relieve the poor animal's pain very quickly.

Jane phoned around the farmers I had arranged to see and told them I wouldn't be there until later in the day, and I set off for Glenlivet.

When I arrived at the farm, Billy's wife Jenny and small son came to the door to greet me. I got Jenny to fill a bucket with warm water as I put on my boots and over-trousers. It was one of those days when the sky is black but every now and then there's a burst of sunlight, making the view across the valley really dramatic.

As I walked up the short hill towards the barn, Billy arrived in the tractor. He's a fit young chap, but it looked as though he'd had a few long nights calving; his face, normally cheerful, was drawn. 'Not a very good way to end this year's calving, George,' he said.

There wasn't any point in saying much; we both knew the score. I know how much it means to any farmer to lose a calf, and there's something frustrating about it being the last one of the batch as well. The cruel hand of fate had turned what promised to be a triumphant moment into a terrible disappointment.

In the barn the black heifer was down on the straw. She had one leg under her body and was lying still. The only movement came as she panted rhythmically with the pain. The body of the dead calf was halfway out of her, its head and forelegs hanging limply.

It's a sight that always depresses me. It's sad that the cow's had to go through all that effort to end up with nothing, and I don't like to see a calf that was never given the chance of life.

Billy helped me move the cow on to her front. We had a bit of a job getting the legs from underneath her so that they stretched out behind her, but Billy's used to pulling animals around and he soon had her as I wanted. I gave the cow a spinal anaesthetic, just like the epidural women are given during childbirth, and while we were waiting for it to take effect Billy helped me on with my calving gown.

Putting it on, I couldn't help comparing this operation with the numerous times I've pulled live calves out over the last weeks. It made the whole situation seem even more poignant. I held the cow's tail to feel how limp it had become, a good gauge of how well the anaesthetic was working. 'She's pretty sick, Billy,' I warned.

'Aye, George, she's had a bad time.' I might have imagined it, but I'm sure that Billy had visibly relaxed over the last few minutes. It was almost as though now I was there he knew that he'd have a brief period when someone else was making the decisions. He got the rope and tied it on to the dead calf's legs. He knew what to do, and pulled the calf as far out as he could. I took my long knife and cut around the calf's body, as close to the cow as possible, being extra careful not to cut the cow in the process. She'd suffered enough as it was.

The exposed half of the dead calf came away and the rest slipped back inside the cow. The next part of the examination would reveal whether I'd been successful in getting enough of the dead calf out in the first cut. The second stage is to put a loop of thin cutting wire inside the cow, slip it over between the hind legs, then use it like a cheese wire to cut the remaining half inside the cow in two. If too much of the calf's body is left inside you can't reach far enough in to put the wire over and that's not an ideal solution for us or the animal.

I felt inside the cow and for a moment thought I wasn't going to be able to reach the back . . . but then I found I could just touch it with my finger tips. A great sense of relief came over me that I'd be able to use the wire. I reached in and just managed to slip it over the hind legs. Then with the wire looped in between the hind legs inside the cow, and the ends of the wire outside, I started a sawing motion, pulling the wire backwards and forwards, gradually cutting the remaining part of the calf in two. It took a lot of effort. I think the mild winter's made me soft – I got out of breath a lot quicker today than last time I did this job.

After a good deal of sawing, the wire came through and I was able to reach in and remove the legs one at a time. 'You can see why it got stuck, George,' Billy said as he examined the pieces. Sure enough it would have been a big brute. He carried on thoughtfully, 'It's the only one I've had problems with from that bull, though.' Usually the farmers know a bull's track record and when it has a tendency to leave large offspring. In this case there wasn't much to put it down to except that it was just one of those freaks of nature.

I gave the cow a final examination. She was all right except for a small nick in the vagina wall, which had been there from the start. 'She looks pretty bad, Billy, but she's got youth on her side,' I said, trying to give him a bit of comfort while I gave the cow a dose of penicillin. I'm sure she'll recover pretty quickly, and Billy will be able to get her back in calf next year. I told him to give her a drink and something to eat later on.

Off came the calving gown, and I saw that my shirt sleeves were covered in blood – clean on this morning as well. There'd be another laundry bill from Jane!

We went back to the house together. 'We've been very lucky this year with the calving,' Billy said as we walked, 'but unfortunately this morning I'm afraid the luck simply ran out.' This was all said in a very matter-of-fact way, with no suggestion of self pity. I went inside to get cleaned up and left Billy to go back to the fields. There's no time to dwell on this sort of thing when you're a working farmer.

TUESDAY 2 MAY

T HERE CAN'T BE many vets in this country who can count reindeer amongst their patients; they are certainly not high on the list of priorities on veterinary courses! I had to learn about them when a herd arrived on the Cairngorms in the early Fifties. A small stocky Swedish man called Mikel Utsi and his six foot tall wife Dr Ethel Lindgren set up an experiment to re-introduce reindeer to Scotland where they had last lived eight hundred years before. I remember Dr Lindgren (who was always called EJ), telling me about their first visit to the Cairngorms in 1947 on holiday. Utsi (he was always called by his surname) had stood looking across the hills and jokingly suggested that they were so like the Arctic conditions reindeer were used to that he thought Cairn Gorm could support a herd. The joke became a reality and a few years later the first members of the herd arrived from Lapland, and were put out to graze on the rugged hillside.

This was all happening at the height of the Cold War and the local lore had it that the project was financed by the Ministry of Defence because they wanted a reservoir of reindeer in case the Russians interfered with the migration of the animals within Lapland. Lapland is partly in northern Russia, partly in Norway, Sweden and Finland, and the reindeer travel across borders constantly. The theory was that the dastardly Russians were determined to grab the reindeer for themselves, and destroy the economy of the area! Implausible as this now sounds in the era of Glasnost, many bar philosophers were convinced that it all made sense. Whether the story was true or not, we all came to think of the herd in the hills as our contribution to the Cold War.

The first time I met EJ was after I'd been up to treat the reindeer with Utsi, and he invited me back for coffee. We went along to the wigwam which they used as a base up on Cairn Gorm, and there was EJ sitting cross-legged on the floor. I was most disappointed when she produced a tin of Nescafé. I suppose I thought she'd have some primitive form of roasted bean. But my disappointment evaporated when she produced a bottle of Swedish Schnapps, which they both insisted was the best in the world. As we sat there in the wigwam I noticed strips of meat being dried in the smoke of the fire. I asked Utsi what they were

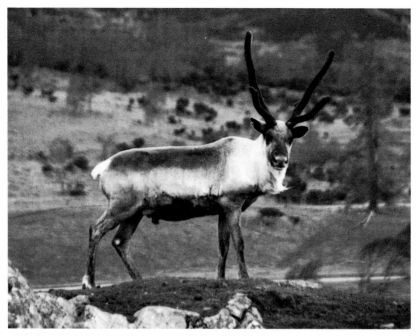

Reindeer on Cairn Gorm

and he dug into the pocket and brought out a lump of something which he'd offered me earlier in the day when we'd been out on the hills. It was reindeer meat which he used as sort of iron rations. It just shows that when you don't know what you're eating you don't mind.

EJ was quite a woman. In the late Twenties she'd led several major explorations into central Asia. She had studied Chinese and experimental psychology at Cambridge and learnt several languages, including Russian and Mongol. It was in China that she became interested in reindeer and through that interest met Utsi who was a Swedish reindeer owner. When all her travelling stopped she devoted herself to looking after the reindeer in the Cairngorms and researching their health and habits.

The reindeer took to their new abode, and began to breed successfully. A few years later EJ was offered a huge contract by a film company to provide the reindeer for a film about Santa Claus. She was offered £300 000 to take a team down to Pinewood Studios to pull the sleigh.

About a year before this was all due to happen, we had to perform a vasectomy on the lead reindeer. He was a vital member of the team, since without him the others wouldn't pull properly. Our operating theatre was a hillside in the Cairngorms, and our operating table the heather. I was a bit worried about doing anything to a potential star, but we had no choice. I used a new anaesthetic which worked a treat – the reindeer was flat out during the operation which proved to be quite tricky. When I finished I expected that he would just about be coming round, but he was *still* flat out. We left him for a few minutes, then gave him a shake. Still no response.

I began to get worried. I could see EJ's £300 000 contract disappearing because the essential member of the team was missing. Leaving Utsi to watch over the unconscious reindeer, I drove off to get some antidote. When I returned I saw the figure of Utsi still hunched over the prone shape in the heather, and assumed the worst. I gave the reindeer the antidote and it was a great relief that before very long he was up on his feet and off, unaware of the anxiety that he'd caused. He recovered from his experience but they were just about to set off when EJ decided that she didn't like the way the film company planned to use the reindeer team and she withdrew from the contract. She wasn't worried about losing the money, but more about the welfare of her charges. In the end the film company had to fly in a team of reindeer from Norway, and some trainers who for some strange reason came from Los Angeles.

I got to know both EJ and Utsi well over the years. There was one evening when old Utsi came to the house to ask for some advice and we sat in the kitchen drinking and talking away. We were very busy at the time and I was so tired that I didn't really listen to what he was going on about, but I do remember hearing something about Canada. When he'd gone Jane, who'd been sitting in one corner listening to the chat, asked me if I realised what I'd agreed to do. I couldn't understand what she meant – as far as I was concerned Utsi had been talking away about his beloved reindeer, and I'd given him a sympathetic ear.

Then she explained that what he'd actually been saying was that he had to go to Canada to try to discover why the reindeer there were dying out, and had asked me to go with him. I'd not been listening to what he was saying, and had just 'yes' every so often, which he took as my firm commitment to become part of his expedition.

I didn't hear any more from him for a while but sure enough

he didn't forget and I had to make all sorts of excuses about being too busy. In the end he took someone else with him. In Canada, Utsi found out that the reindeer were being killed for food by the very Eskimos who were being paid to look after them.

Utsi died back in 1979, but EJ carried on the work with the herd until she died a year ago at the age of eighty-three. The herd is now run by Alan and Tilly Smith as a scientific experiment and a tourist attraction, and Alan phoned this morning and asked me to have a look at one of the herd who's having trouble eating. They've had a few problems with litter left lying around by tourists at the bottom of one of the chairlifts on Cairn Gorm. The animals see this colourful stuff and eat it, sometimes with fatal consequences – in fact they've lost three of the herd during the last year.

Alan thinks that another one has got something stuck in her throat and wants me to see if I can do anything to save it. It makes me really angry that visitors come up here and treat the place like they would their own cities, dropping litter everywhere and leaving tin cans lying around to cause damage and pain to animals.

The herd lives quite high up and the winds fair whistle around, but I wasn't prepared for the gale that greeted us as we left the warmth of the car. Even though it was May the wind was howling around us, and a mixture of rain and sleet searched out even the smallest gap in our clothing. High on the hills, the wind chills you to the bones very quickly, and I cursed myself for not wearing warmer clothes.

We left the car and straightaway the first problem occurred. The bag holding the feed blew away in the strong wind, scattering food across the barren hillside. Alan ran after it, and managed to rescue the bag and salvage some of the contents. We had to hope that enough would remain to entice the herd towards us. If this didn't work we would face a chase across the hill which would almost inevitably lead to the failure of our mission.

In the distance, through the walls of driving rain, I could just see the herd, well camouflaged on the hillside. We scrabbled down a small valley, me holding on to my Gladstone bag, Alan dragging the remains of the feed bag. When we got to the bottom of the valley we had to cross a stream, swollen by the recent rains. Alan crossed with no difficulty. I put one foot on a rock which seemed an ideal stepping stone, and the other … well I'd like to say that it went firmly on to dry ground on the other bank. In fact the gleeful cry from Alan, 'The vet's up to his waist in it again!' describes the situation perfectly.

I couldn't print my comments. Suffice to say I was thankful that the only witnesses were the reindeer and Alan! Trudging forward with squelching wellingtons and clothes which now felt more like a set of sponges, we moved at a snail's pace towards the herd. As we reached them Alan shook out the meagre contents of the food bag. Fortunately it contained enough to convince them that it was the first course of a gourmet meal. They lined up on either side of the improvised banquet and concentrated on eating.

Alan pointed out the one with the problem. He moved around the head of the line and grabbed at a leg. I was next to him by then and in one swift move had the other leg in my grasp, and we had her. Alan lay on the reindeer as I opened my bag to prepare the jaw expanders, an instrument more commonly used on dogs' teeth to keep the mouth open while we examine the mouth or throat. In the cold, driving rain my hands were soon nearing numbness, and I knew that the race was on to beat the elements. The expanders slipped frequently – without the long canine teeth which they were designed for they had nothing to grip on. With the light failing I had difficulty in seeing inside the reindeer's mouth, and the wind blew so hard that we could hardly hear each other talking, even though we were standing a few feet apart.

I told Alan to hold the reindeer's tongue, so that I could look inside her mouth. I could see blood at the back of the throat, but no sign of any obstruction. I knew if there was anything there I had to find it. Another day unable to eat could make this one reindeer which wouldn't be pulling Santa's sleigh at Christmas!

The rain and wind had really penetrated my whole body by now but just at the point when my hands resembled blocks of ice, I saw a tiny glint in the throat. It was a great feeling. Now all I had to do was operate the long forceps. The damage to the throat was obvious, and I reached gently down to the edge of the shining metal and manoeuvred the instrument around it. The offending article had lodged itself into the walls of the throat and the only option was a gentle tug to remove it. The pull overcame the resistance and the throat released its damaging contents: a metal disc about $2\frac{1}{2}$ inches across.

'By God, it's another tin can!' Alan's shout was so loud that it carried above the howling gale, and his anger was obvious even

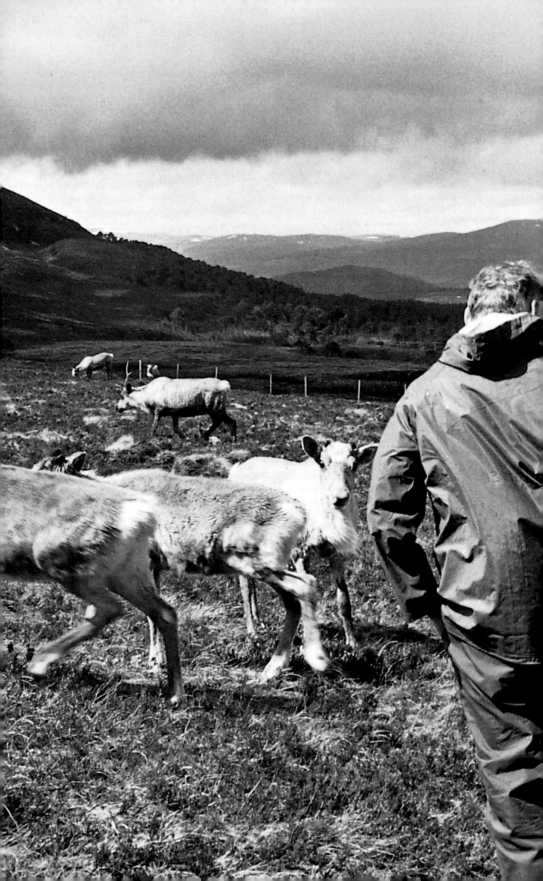

though by now we both looked like drowned rats. I gave the poor beast a shot of penicillin to stop any infection. It took a great mental push to load the syringe and inject the animal, which was still lying quietly under Alan's weight. As soon as the injection had been delivered we let the animal get up and it was off with no ill effects to join the rest of the herd. By the time we finished the red noses definitely belonged to us, not the reindeer!

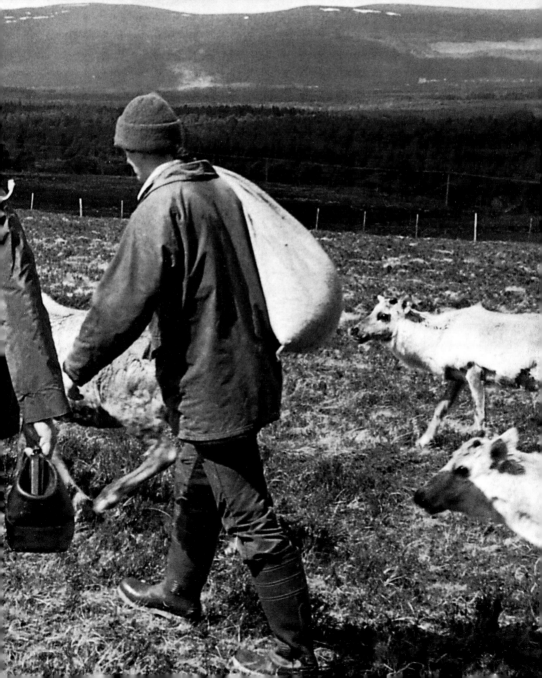

WEDNESDAY 10 MAY

I'M TAKING MY annual holiday tomorrow; I'm going over to the Western Isle of Lewis for a couple of days to lecture to the crofters on sheep fertility. I've done the trip a few times before – it's usually a good laugh, and I hope some use to them.

The great thing about living in a small community like ours up here is that we all try to help each other out. There's a farmer's wife, Jessie Campbell, who originally came from Lewis and her parents still live there. She heard that I'm going, and asked me to take a parcel over for them. I think it means a lot for the old folk to hear a bit of news of their daughter and family from someone who knows them, and can talk about what's going on in their lives, especially when they're living so far away, so I called on Jessie this morning and picked up the parcel.

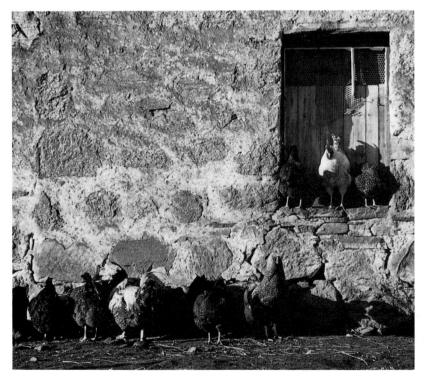

A typical welcoming party.

FRIDAY 12 MAY

I'M SITTING IN the airport lounge at Stornoway on Lewis waiting for the plane to take me back to Inverness. It was a great couple of days, I think my talk went well and certainly the wee ceilidh we had last night was great fun. The trip nearly got off to a bad start, mind you. It was five thirty in the morning and I was about to drive away from home when Jane came running out with the parcel for Jessie's mum and dad. I almost forgot to take it with me. It's a good job Jane knows what's going on; I'd forever be forgetting things else.

When I arrived in Stornoway it was a beautiful, bright day. The clear blue sky and strong sun belied the bitterness of the icy winds. Inside the terminal building the usual envelope was waiting for me on the notice-board. It's become a sort of ritual that they leave the hire car keys for me in that way.

I drove off to see the MacDonalds and when I arrived, Ian, Jessie's brother, was busy making tweed. Most of the crofters' income in that part of the island is from weaving cloth in the traditional way on hand looms. They aren't allowed to be mechanised if they want it to be called Harris tweed.

Ian stopped his work and we went into the house. After a warm greeting from Mr and Mrs MacDonald senior, I gave them Jessie's parcel. Mrs MacDonald took the brown box, thanked me and put it to one side. 'I didn't think it was the right shape,' I said, 'so I brought you this wee sample of local Strathspey produce as well.' I unzipped my coat. 'I hid it inside here in case the neighbours saw me arriving with it.'

I reached in and pulled out a bottle of my favourite whisky, Tamnavulin. Mrs Macdonald gave me a playful thump on my arm in thanks. 'Well, we should sample it straight away, I think,' said Mr Macdonald, 'just in case the journey's ruined it.'

We moved through to their front room and chatted away over a dram and cakes. They wanted to know all about how Jessie was getting on. 'I saw her yesterday and she's looking great,' I said. 'Just like whisky, she improves with age.'

'Well, none of us are getting any younger.' Mrs MacDonald laughed. 'It's only the dead who don't grow older, isn't it?'

It's always great to meet people like these, with a good hearty sense of humour and fun. I asked Ian if he'd not found himself a wife yet. He said that he was still looking. 'You need a working wife, Ian,' I told him. He nodded in agreement. 'But they're kind of scarce these days, you know.'

Ian smiled, not quite sure whether to take my pronouncements seriously or not. 'You marry them for their beauty and keep them for their usefulness!' I continued.

Crofts like the MacDonalds' are strips of land about twice the width of a house which run in parallel plots away from the seashore. There's just enough land to graze a few cattle and sheep, and many of them have a building with a loom in it.

We talked for a while about the change in agriculture on the island. You always used to see cows grazing everywhere. The wives would milk them by hand and rear the calf. I think it's probably too much hard work for the people these days. 'We used to have plenty butter then,' said Mrs MacDonald, in a slightly nostalgic tone, 'and cream as well.'

This is one of the interesting things about the lifestyle of farming people like these. Here they are, having spent their lives eating and drinking everything we're told is bad for us today, and seemingly not suffering at all. I asked them what they reckoned to all the new thinking on health. 'Well as long as you get plenty hard work,' said Mr MacDonald, 'you can eat anything.'

'Our doctor back in Grantown says that you'll be all right as long as you're short of breath twice a day,' I said. 'But not from passion!' They murmured agreement.

Having put the world to rights, I left them to their work and made my way across the island to the place where I was to give my talk. I stopped on the way to get a brief lungful of sea air. The air was alive with that freshness you get when the waves rolling in make the shoreline a seething spectacle of frothing white water. All around me on the cliffs was a carpet of wild flowers, and there was not a single person to be seen.

I THOUGHT ABOUT the last time I'd been involved in one of these Agricultural Training Board visits. It turned out to be the only time in my life that I've had to work on a human being. I was on the island of Muck, and one of the chaps coming to the course fell off his bicycle, and split his head open just above the eye. I had a look at him and decided that he really ought to have stitches, so we phoned the local doctor, who was on the neighbouring island of Eigg. He said that the chap would need to get stitched up at the Belford Hospital at Fort William. That would have meant getting the launch out from Arisaig specially, so the chap asked me if I would stitch him up.

By a strange quirk of medical ethics, we veterinary surgeons are allowed to treat humans, but doctors aren't allowed near our patients. And I happened to have a set of stitching equipment with me. It wasn't really designed for use in this sort of emergency – I'd intended to use it as part of my talk to demonstrate how to stitch up sheep after they've given birth, which has to be done sometimes. However, since it was all I had available it had to do. I just gave him the local anaesthetic I would normally give to sheep, and started work on him right there. His fellow crofters had come to hear me talking about lambing, but seemed quite happy to watch this different form of medical operation instead.

I was surprised to discover how tough his skin was. It was more difficult to get a needle through him that it would have been on a similar-sized animal. I finished the stitching, which wasn't vastly different from any other type of stitching, except that normally my patients don't attempt to carry on a conversation while I work. Then came a more difficult request. He'd hurt his shoulder as well and asked me to look at that, which of course I did. I said that I was pretty sure that it wasn't dislocated, but I have to say that I wasn't all that good at examining him. I think if he'd been on all fours it would have been different.

However, the next day they decided to be on the safe side, and that it was enough of a medical emergency to call for the launch. It came out and took him over to the mainland. I heard later that the surgeon in Fort William had a look at him and asked him who had stitched him up. 'The vet,' he replied.

I think it took the surgeon a bit by surprise. He was kind enough to joke that, 'they're not all the butchers we think they are, then!' and say that I'd actually done a good job. I think he must have been surprised that I even vaguely knew what I was doing. They left the stitches in anyway.

I WAS HOPEFUL that nothing as exciting would present itself for my attention on this course. My Gladstone bag didn't contain stitching gear in any case – only my overnight essentials and some teaching aids, which had been collected from Grantown's slaughterhouse the previous day. When I arrived at the Crofters'

Union building there were a few cattle trailers outside. Inside there were half-a-dozen tups in behind some crating, and about twenty men and women chatting away. Carla, who organises the courses, welcomed me and we started the course straight away.

They'd asked me to talk about fertility in rams, or tups as we call them in Strathspey. Tups often get neglected and they don't work well when their time comes. If the farmers have a few simple pieces of knowledge, it can make a great deal of difference to how their tups perform. One of the things we find is that farmers spend a lot of money on a new tup which they put out in the field. Straight away the other tups attack it, and break its neck. I think the best solution is to put all the tups into a small pen with no food for a couple of days. Then they've no room to back off, run at one another and break each other's necks. After a couple of days when they're let out to graze, they're too hungry to be bothered about charging the new boy. This advice was listened to and seemed to be welcomed.

As I'd been talking I'd been fiddling around inside my bag trying to take out my teaching props – a polythene bag full of tups' testicles – without revealing my pyjamas. It was no good, I had to remove my night attire from the bag first. This brought a round of smiles, and the comment, 'That's very appropriate,' from one of the crofters. I laid the sexual organs out on the bench in front of me, and started to run through the anatomy of the animal.

Tups have some of the largest testicles for their body size of any animal I know. There's a story in Grantown of a Suffolk tup getting loose in a field of sheep, where he served thirty ewes in one day. They knew it had to be him because he was the only Suffolk tup in the area and they leave distinctive black-headed lambs. I described the working parts that lay in front of me, and showed the crofters how to tell when they bought a tup if it was in full working order. It's very easy to tell, just by feeling, if there's anything basic wrong with an animal, but it's the sort of thing that many farmers don't know. This course was intended to give them enough experience to be able to spot a dud at market.

Then I turned to the penis. It's a quite remarkable breeding machine, with a thing on the end of it called a worm. When the tup serves, this worm whirls about inside the ewe and helps to spread the semen all around. Unfortunately the one I had brought so carefully over that morning on the plane had had its worm cut off by Raymond at the slaughterhouse!

THE CROFTERS CERTAINLY seemed to have picked up the ability to examine the animals after my instruction, which was gratifying. As I was packing up my anatomical samples, one of them asked if I'd like to go back for a few drinks. I noticed that there wasn't any question of the niceties of 'a drink'. You were invited for 'a few drinks' and you knew that was exactly what you were going to have.

It turned into a real ceilidh. There was a man in one corner with a fiddle, playing traditional tunes. I suppose about twenty of us crammed into the front room of the house. With the golden liquid flowing, and the gentle lilting sounds from the fiddle, it was great to just sit back, glass in hand, and listen and talk into the wee, small hours and beyond. I discovered that the man sitting next to me had been engaged to a woman in the room for twenty years – they obviously didn't want to rush into anything.

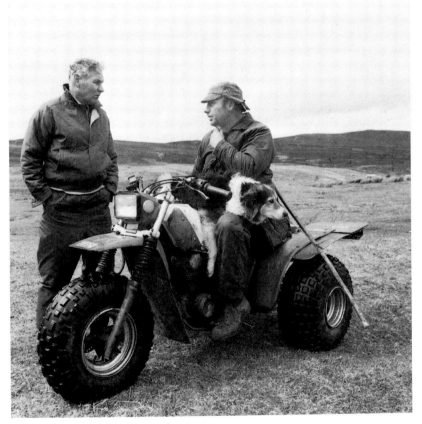

In conversation with a modern shepherd.

TUESDAY 6 JUNE

I LEFT THE HOUSE this morning knowing that the outcome of my first call was likely to be an unsatisfactory one. The phone call I'd received from Mrs Watson was not very encouraging.

We'd first got involved the night before when Willie went over to Glentromie to see a horse which had what we thought was colic. We had every hope that we would be able to do something for it, but the latest news was not good. One of the snags of a district like this is that some of the patients are a long way away and this particular emergency was over 23 miles to the west, out past Aviemore and beyond Loch Insch. That meant another day's routine work out the window, but then if I'd wanted a nine to five job I wouldn't have chosen this one!

On the long drives I invariably run through all the possibilities I might be confronted with on arrival. One of the complications which horses with colic suffer from up here in the northeast of Scotland is Grass Sickness. The problem is that no one really knows what causes it or how to treat it, consequently it's almost always fatal. Alternatively it may have been simple spasmodic colic, basically wind, caused by something in the food. Sadly, though, it sounds as though this particular case could be a twisted bowel. If worse came to worst I had the humane killer with me, a point 22 gun which we use to put down large animals. Not a job I like doing, especially with horses.

I think most people in all walks of life would agree that the day you get complacent about your duties is the day to give up. The clinical condition of any particular animal may be something which I've seen a thousand times before, but the location or the owner's attitude or lack of facilities can lead to a whole different set of problems which in turn can affect the way in which treatment is dispensed. I already knew that there was an added difficulty in this case. The owner of the horse lives in the south of England and I knew that I might have to take the decision myself without being able to consult her.

The stables where the horse is kept are away in a valley. The surrounding hills were shrouded in mist when I arrived. As I drove across the white-fenced bridge which crossed the River Tromie I saw the stable block in the distance with three white ponies in the yard, and the two figures of the groom, Mrs Watson, and her teenage son Gavin. As I drove up I could see a fourth pony rolling around on its back in the mud. There was no need to ask which one was in need of my attention.

This first sight of the animal did not encourage optimism. When horses and ponies are in pain they often roll on their backs in an attempt to release some of the tension. Getting out of the car I put my stethoscope in my pocket and joined the two people standing quietly studying the animal.

'Morning, Mrs Watson. How are you today?'

'Not too bad considering all this.' The strain of what must have been a worrying few hours showed on her face and in her slightly stooped stance. One of the problems with looking after other people's animals is that when something goes wrong it's often harder to reconcile yourself than when it's your own. I asked Gavin to put a head collar on the horse and hold her still for me.

The process of elimination began. I listened to her heart with the stethoscope. A moment or two of intense concentration, as much a chance for me to think as to learn more about the illness of the horse. Then I took her temperature.

'Her temperature's way up, which isn't a good sign really.' I knew that the more gentle warnings I could give of what I feared was going to be necessary, the better.

'Has she been lying down like this for long?' I asked as I continued the examination.

'She was all right when I saw her early this morning, but when I came up here later she was lying on her back, obviously in pain.' Mrs Watson was gently stroking the horse's nose in a soft, comforting way. I asked if she'd had any change in her feed.

Mrs Watson paused, and I could see her going over in her mind any change in routine. 'No, none at all.'

'I only ask because sometimes it can cause problems, but I don't think it's anything like that in any case.' Although I needed to cover all possibilities, I didn't want her thinking that she'd done something to cause the illness.

'I'd like to have a feel inside her and see if I can tell what's wrong.' I asked Gavin to lead the horse into the stable.

'There's not much light inside there.' Mrs Watson said.

'Don't worry,' I smiled gently, 'it's pretty dark inside her.'

By the time I returned from the car with my bucket of warm

water the horse was tied up inside the stable. 'Mum's gone down to get her boots on,' said Gavin.

I knew that I really should have waited until she returned to hold up the foreleg to stop the horse kicking me as I gave her an internal examination, but I didn't want to delay any longer than absolutely necessary. I didn't think the boy would be strong enough on his own so I resigned myself to the thought that I'm well insured and at least he could pick up the pieces if I was kicked through the window at great speed! Having soaped my arm I worked it gently deep inside my patient and carefully felt around. I remember the first time I did this sort of examination not being able to discern the various parts as easily as the nice neat diagrams in the book had suggested I would. It was more like putting my hand inside one of my mother's dumplings! But it's one of those practical skills you suddenly find you've acquired and can use with no difficulty. I suppose it's a bit like the first time you get the hang of riding a two wheeled bike.

Mrs Watson had been right, it was dark inside the stable but I could see the boy's face as he stroked the horse. He was obviously a sensitive young chap and this whole ordeal was telling on him, despite which he was being strong.

I felt what I feared I would find, but I withdrew my arm, resoaped it and had a second examination. I was sure that my diagnosis was correct, so I couldn't put off imparting the result any longer. 'I'm afraid she's got a twisted bowel, and there's nothing we can do about it.'

'How would she get that?' Mrs Watson seemed to take the news as though she'd expected it.

'It's just one of those things which happens sometimes to horses.'

Both mother and son were now stroking the pony with real affection and I could see that they were very upset. 'She's in a lot of pain, anyhow.' The mother spoke in a low, quiet voice.

I explained that she was certainly going to die, and reinforced the fact that there was no hope. If she'd been near a veterinary hospital then maybe we could have done something, operated on her, perhaps, but even then just getting her there would have killed her. I didn't add that even if she survived a journey the chances of surviving an operation which could cost over a thousand pounds would probably be no greater than one in ten. In this practice we don't have any facilities for doing that kind of work because the cost of providing them is astronomically high, and would just be impractical for us.

'I'll take on the responsibility for putting her down,' I said. 'I'm sure Mrs Hone would want it. She can give me a ring if she wants me to explain it all to her.'

I explained that we'd take her outside where the knackery could get to her easily. Mrs Watson showed signs of being uncomfortable. 'Will they come today? My daughter will be in from school. One of the other ponies is hers so she always comes up to look at them and she'll be very upset.'

This was one of those extra unexpected problems which complicate matters. I thought that I could probably persuade the knackery man, Mr Murphy, to come out even though they are 70-odd miles in the other direction. They're very good when they know there's a problem like that, but I knew it would probably need me to call up a favour! 'I'll give them a ring and see what they can do.' I wanted to relieve her of as much stress as possible, especially because the next thing was to ask how she wanted to put the pony down. I always like to give the owner (or in this case the person responsible), the choice of either shooting or injection. Sometimes with a horse which is excited, the injection can cause problems. Mrs Watson didn't really even have to think, straight away she replied that she'd like it injected.

Gavin led the horse outside, past my car, to a patch of ground where the knackery lorry would be able to get to it easily. Although it was obvious that he was moved by the pony's plight, he was doing everything asked of him as efficiently as anyone could have done. I thought that he was the sort of boy who would really grow up to be an asset to his family, the right mixture of compassion and strength. I suppose it's the sort of training you get when you live in the country and deal with life-and-death matters every day from an early age.

As I opened the boot of the car to prepare the injection I mused on one of the paradoxes of veterinary life. A lot of our work involves putting down animals which are suffering, and you know it really is one of the most useful things we do in many ways. We use a drug called Euthatol which is a highly concentrated anaesthetic. As always in these situations I hoped that I'd find the vein first time so that it would go smoothly, for animal and humans alike.

As I walked over to the pony which was standing quietly I

noticed Mrs Watson had wandered over to the other ponies who were looking over towards our group. As she stood there stroking each of their noses in turn it was almost as though they were saying farewell to their companion. Even from that distance I could see that her face was wet from tears.

'Right, son, if you just hold its head round that way a wee bit.' Although the young boy showed signs of tension, he simply did as asked. I could see that he was steeling himself to do exactly what he was told as precisely as possible.

I jabbed the needle in and the drops of blood which came out showed that I'd hit the vein. As I connected the syringe I gave the final instructions. 'If it starts to stagger you just let go.'

I gave the injection and the pony reacted almost immediately. Gavin was watching the animal intently, so I had to shout. 'Now out of the road, son, let it go.' I was afraid that he might get caught under the horse as it fell, but he was well out of the way by the time it hit the ground.

The pony gave a few last deep sighs and it was all over.

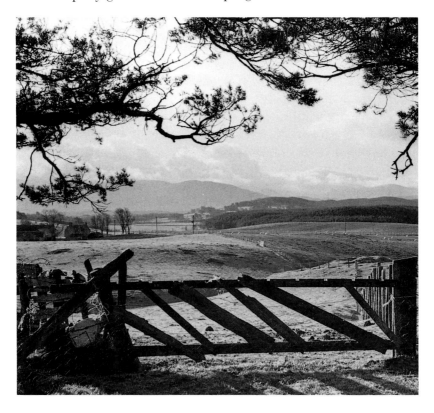

Thursday 6 July

S INCE I STARTED to write this erratic diary my thoughts have turned to many of the old characters who were scattered around the area, and who used to be part of our practice.

This morning when I was driving along the road from Tomintoul down Glen Livet to Grantown I passed the track which led to Lagual, a remote farm which was run by a very odd couple.

They were two brothers, Roland and Sidney Gordon, both thickset and dark, big strong chaps who were used to hard work all their days. Roland was the older of the two and and the brains of the outfit. Sidney was more reserved and lived very much in Roland's shadow. They stayed together in the same farmhouse, spent their days together in the same fields and barns, and yet they never spoke to each other. In fact there were very few people in the area who'd heard them talk at all.

There was a cattle sale in Tomintoul twice a year. It really was a social occasion, a great day out for all the farmers of the district. This was long before all-day opening hours were brought in, but the local pubs had special licences to open for the duration of the sale. It wasn't surprising, therefore, to find many of the farmers in the local hostelries during the proceedings, and long after, getting a bit tight. In fact it got to be such a good day out that it became a real bone of contention in some families. One year one farmer's wife got so fed up with trying to drag her husband out of the pub that when it got late into the night, well after closing time, she telephoned the police and told them that there was out of hours drinking going on, so that they were forced to go along and chuck them all out. So for most farmers this was a real day to look forward to. But not for the brothers Gordon.

In order to get their sheep to market most farmers would hire a cattle float, a truck, but Roland and Sidney would drive their animals the 5 miles over the hills to Tomintoul. Even going back twenty years that was a really outdated method. As soon as they had put all their stock into the appropriate pens, without a word passing between them, Sidney would turn round and walk back across the fields.

The brothers' silent relationship was a bit like those monks who've taken a vow of silence. I would often see them working at their turnips, but on opposite sides of the field. It would be wrong to say that they never argued, because they never spoke, yet in their own way they got on really well. They were never nasty to one another in their demeanour.

They were devout Catholics, staunch chapel-goers. One Sunday when the clocks went back, Sidney was seen walking across the fields to go to church. He'd obviously forgotten to reset his watch because he was an hour too early. An hour later his brother was seen walking across the fields. Even though they lived in the same house and Roland would have seen his brother getting dressed ready for church, he didn't say anything. There would have been no malice in his actions or lack of them, though – it was just the way they lived their lives. I visit so many homes that I can tell straight away by now when there's some sort of atmosphere, and there was none there.

I came into contact with them every year on my annual visit to them to test their cattle. People who live out in the wilds of nowhere on remote crofts and farms were usually very glad to see folk to have a chat and blather away to. So much so that I would usually try and allow a few extra minutes just to sit and talk after the work was done. But Roland and Sidney were very different. They would never speak unless you spoke to them directly, and they'd certainly never carry on a conversation.

I regarded them as a bit of a challenge, I suppose. I used to keep asking questions so that they had to answer. Being naturally polite like most country folk, they would reply, but you'd have to ask another question before they'd say anything else. Their answers were not exactly monosyllabic but as near as they could be while still being polite. To say they were men of few words would be to make them sound too eloquent.

I can remember one annual visit when the conversation went something like this:

'Have you had anyone here since I was here last year?'

'Yes.'

'Who was that?'

'The income tax man.'

'What did he come for?'

'To sort out our tax.'

On a very rare occasion, one year I had to make a second visit to calve a cow. It was in the depths of winter and the snow

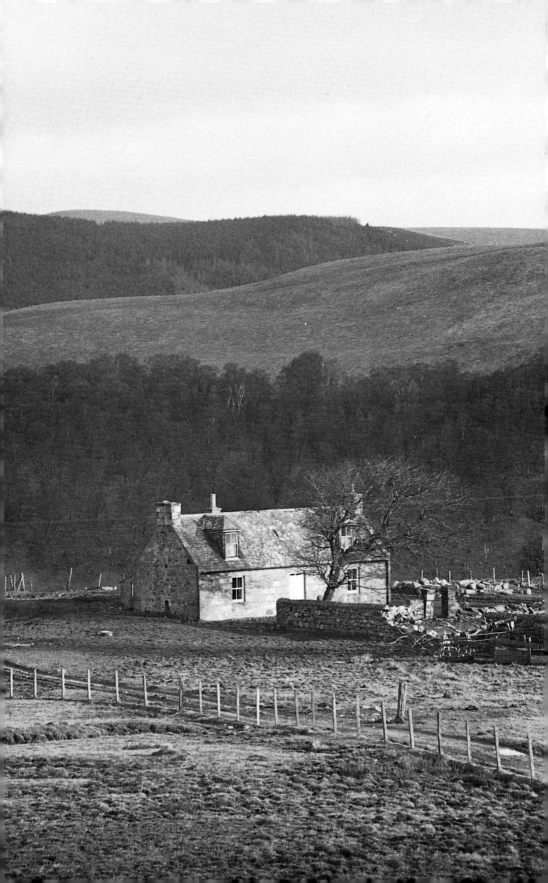

was so thick and deep that I had to leave my car miles away at the Pole Inn, and tramp across the fields to get to the farm. I think I must have been fit in those days! I called in at the Bochel, another local farm where the farmer was Charlie Grant, always known in the local way as Charlie Bochel. He was a really nice chap and offered to come and help. So off we trudged into the snow. On arrival we were greeted with nothing more than a nod.

Undeterred we set about calving the cow. It was quite amazing really that during the whole process there wasn't a word from either brother's lips. I admit I was really annoyed on Charlie's behalf, but I suppose it was just their way. I'm sure it wasn't deliberate rudeness on their part, and, looking back, I know that they appreciated what we'd done.

The only time Sidney went away further than the Tomintoul market was to see his brother in hospital when he was dying from cancer. The trip to Dufftown was the first time he'd seen a railway. He really led a sheltered life.

There was a case of sheep worrying in the district just after Roland died. The policeman got the job of going around all the farms and asking them if they'd had their dogs shut in, to see if he could find out whose dogs had caused the problems. He went to Lagual to see about the farm dogs, and Sidney opened the door and stood there like a dummy.

The bobby was taken aback at this tall man who didn't say anything, so as a form of address in his deep Scots voice, he said, 'Well, how's the man?'

And with hardly a flicker Sidney replied in an equally deep gruff Scots voice, 'He's dead.' He never considered himself to be the man of the house, even when his brother had passed on!

One day the postie went there to deliver some mail, quite a rarity in its own right. He noticed that no one was around and went round the back to check that Sidney was all right. Looking in a window, he saw Sidney's body inside lying on the floor. He phoned the policeman, who in turn got hold of the bank manager. For some reason he thought that there might be money in the house.

They eventually broke in and removed the body. When they started to look around, the policeman opened a drawer and over £9000 in pound notes came tumbling out. Twenty years ago that was a lot of money.

Today their farm is a holiday home.

TUESDAY 1 AUGUST

SITTING IN THE front room leafing through this diary, I noticed that it was almost exactly a year ago that I started writing it. The timing is appropriate because next week is the annual Grantown Show, which is to Strathspey what the World Snooker Championships Final is to Steve Davis. As ever, we're hopeful that a good number of our clients will be among the winners in the various categories. It's great to see animals which you've treated winning a prize; it gives us great professional pride and personal pleasure. It's always good to have a cause to celebrate in the beer tents, although we have been known to manage the odd drink in there without a specific reason.

Once Grantown Show is past we'll embark on a new farming year, and the cycle will start again. The past twelve months have certainly been interesting. We were blessed by the mildest winter that anyone in the district can remember. The weather was kind to us and the farmers, although it did give rise to an outbreak of disease among the newly born calves, which was brought on by the warm weather helping germs breed.

Neil, our new assistant vet, has settled in, and I have every hope that he'll stay for another year at least. Much as I've moaned about the television people coming up and getting in our way, I suppose we've enjoyed the experience on the whole. One thing they've done for me is open my eyes to the scenery, which I had completely forgotten to notice as I flew through the district thinking about work. If any of us had the slightest aspirations to be television stars, they've disappeared and we're now dreading seeing ourselves on the screen.

Writing this diary has been a good excuse to look back at the last forty years. I've especially enjoyed recalling some of the old characters who used to be so much part of the district. There are fewer and fewer left as the years pass, and I think it's important to remember them – after all they're part of our heritage. It may just be me getting old but as I head for what is usually considered the age to hang up the stethoscope, I feel sure that people are more inhibited these days, more anxious to conform to what society feels is normal. I'm certain that we had more fun in years past, because there weren't so many rules and regulations restricting all aspects of life in general.

I was talking to a farmer today about preparing for another new farming cycle. He said that he always felt that he ought to make a wish for luck, and he wondered what I would ask for if I could have any wish granted. It was an easy one to answer. I told him that I hoped to remain fit to continue my work as I have done the last forty years.

He then asked when I was going to retire. I replied as I have done on many similar occasions. I'll stop when my clients say it's time I retired. So far they're too polite to tell me.

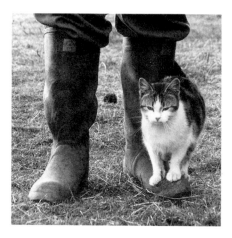